JOHNS HOPKINS
MEDICINE

Dear Readers:

Each year, the Vision White Paper reports on the most exciting advances and the most useful, current information to help you prevent or treat eye disease.

We would like to take this opportunity to explain the various components of this White Paper. The main text provides a thorough overview of what the medical field knows about cataracts, glaucoma, age-related macular degeneration, and diabetic retinopathy—their causes, symptoms, diagnostic procedures, and treatment options. The research columns (located in the margins) report on the latest studies—sometimes confirming what we already know about vision disorders, and sometimes questioning our practices and current understanding (as the scientific process so often does). Finally, the dozen or so features (articles located in shaded boxes throughout the White Paper) focus on special topics that we felt warranted particular attention this year.

Here are some of the feature highlights for 2006:

- The role of **genetics** in eye disease.(page 7)
- **Custom-made vision corrections** by way of new intraocular lenses. (page 13)
- Vision and **Alzheimer's disease**—the problem may not be your eyes. (page 10)
- Preventing the progression of **age-related macular degeneration**. (page 32)
- **New drugs** for fighting **glaucoma**. (page 19)
- Eight **herbs and supplements** that can harm your eyes. (page 40)
- **Macugen**—the latest drug for treating macular degeneration. (page 39)
- **High blood pressure** can threaten your vision. (page 45)
- **Artificial vision**: new frontiers in sight. (page 49)

I hope the information provided in this White Paper will be helpful in educating and guiding anyone affected by eye disease.

Sincerely,

Andrew P. Schachat, M.D.
Professor
Department of Ophthalmology
Johns Hopkins University School of Medicine

AF853346

P. S. Please visit www.HopkinsVision.com for the latest news on eye diseases and other information that will complement your Johns Hopkins White Paper.

THE AUTHORS

Andrew P. Schachat, M.D., graduated from Princeton University and the Johns Hopkins University School of Medicine. He did his ophthalmology residency at the Wilmer Eye Institute at Johns Hopkins Hospital and a vitreoretinal and oncology fellowship at the Wills Eye Hospital in Philadelphia. Currently, he is the Karl Hagen Professor of Ophthalmology and director of the Retinal Vascular Center and the Ocular Oncology Service at the Wilmer Eye Institute. In addition, he is the editor of *Ophthalmology* and is on the editorial board of *The Johns Hopkins Medical Letter: Health After 50*. Dr. Schachat is also the editor of the first two volumes of Steven Ryan's *Retina,* a three-volume textbook of retinal disease for ophthalmologists. He was a principal investigator on the Macular Photocoagulation Study, which proved the benefit of laser treatment for some patients with age-related macular degeneration, and, more recently, on the trials showing the safety and efficacy of photodynamic therapy with verteporfin.

▪ ▪ ▪

Harry A. Quigley, M.D., is the A. Edward Maumenee Professor of Ophthalmology and the director of both the Glaucoma Service and the Dana Center for Preventive Ophthalmology at the Wilmer Eye Institute at Johns Hopkins Hospital. He was a founding member of the American Glaucoma Society and served as its secretary for eight years. He was elected chief executive officer of the Association for Research in Vision and Ophthalmology and editor-in-chief of *Investigative Ophthalmology and Visual Science.*

▪ ▪ ▪

Oliver D. Schein, M.D., M.P.H., is the Burton E. Grossman Professor of Ophthalmology at the Wilmer Eye Institute and carries a joint appointment in the department of epidemiology at the Johns Hopkins University School of Hygiene and Public Health. Dr. Schein's clinical expertise is in medical and surgical conditions of the anterior segment of the eye involving cataracts and complications of cataract surgery, corneal scarring, and corneal surgery. He is an author of the American Academy of Ophthalmology's "Preferred Practice Pattern" on Cataract.

VISION

Andrew P. Schachat, M.D.,

Harry A. Quigley, M.D.,

and

Oliver D. Schein, M.D., M.P.H.

CONTENTS

VISION

The most common eye diseases in people over age 50 are cataracts, glaucoma, age-related macular degeneration, and diabetic retinopathy. Fortunately, if you have one of these eye disorders and are treated early enough, the progression of disease can often be slowed or even halted, helping you return to daily activities such as driving, grocery shopping, reading, and performing household tasks. In addition to medication and surgery, you can take steps on your own to make it easier to live with an eye disorder. A wide array of low vision aids is also available to enhance your vision.

Because most eye disorders cause no symptoms in their early stages, many people are unaware when one first develops. Surveys by researchers at Johns Hopkins have found that about one third of people with an eye disease were unaware of it prior to receiving their diagnosis, and over one third of those between the ages of 65 and 84 years had not visited an ophthalmologist (eye doctor) during the previous year. Periodic visits to an eye care specialist are vital for detecting conditions early enough to allow for effective treatment. Regular check-ups are particularly important if you are over age 65, have a risk factor (especially diabetes) for a serious eye disease, or are in fair or poor general health.

ANATOMY OF THE EYE

The eye is a complex structure that sends nerve impulses to the brain when stimulated by light rays reflected from an object. The brain then processes these impulses to create the perception of vision.

The eye is made up of numerous parts that work together to make vision possible (see the illustration on page 3) . The **iris,** the colored circle in the middle of the eye, is the eye's most prominent structure. The iris is composed of smooth muscles that contract and expand to alter the size of the pupil and control the amount of light that enters the eye. Also visible from the front of the eye is the **pupil**, the opening in the center of the iris that resembles a large black dot. The **sclera**, which makes up part of the outer layer of the eye, is the tough, white connective tissue that covers and protects the majority of the eye.

Also at the front of the eye are the cornea, lens, and conjunctiva. The **cornea** is a transparent, dome-shaped disk that covers the iris and pupil. Beneath the cornea is a transparent, elastic structure called the **lens.** The cornea does about three quarters of the work of focusing light on the retina; the lens does the rest. The **conjunctiva** is a thin, lubricating mucous membrane that covers the sclera and lines the inside of the eyelids.

Inside the sclera lie two more layers. The middle layer, the **choroid**, contains a dark pigment that minimizes scattering of light inside the eye. It is rich in blood vessels that supply nutrients to the **retina**, the innermost layer of the eye that consists of light-sensitive nerve tissue. The retina functions like film in a camera, receiving an imprint of an image and sending it via the optic nerve to the brain to be "developed." The **macula**, at the center of the retina, is a small area responsible for central vision and for seeing detail and color.

The **vitreous humor** is a thick, gel-like substance that fills the back of the eyeball behind the lens. The **aqueous humor** is a watery fluid located in front of the lens. Along with the vitreous humor, the aqueous humor maintains intraocular pressure (the internal pressure of the eye), which is needed to prevent the eyeball from collapsing. Intraocular pressure is controlled by specialized cells that produce aqueous humor and by ducts and canals that drain this fluid from the eye.

REFRACTIVE ERRORS

The major role of the lens is to refract and focus light from both distant and near objects. This is achieved by changes in the shape of the lens. To see at a distance, muscle fibers attached to the lens tighten to flatten the shape of the lens and focus light coming from a distance onto the retina. For close vision, these muscle fibers relax, and the lens reverts to its naturally rounder shape, which focuses light from close objects onto the retina. This process is known as accommodation.

Refractive errors are caused by a deviation in the way light focuses on the retina. The 4 types of refractive errors are nearsightedness (myopia), farsightedness (hyperopia), astigmatism, and presbyopia. All 4 conditions can be corrected with eyeglasses or contact lenses. An increasingly popular alternative to glasses and contacts, especially for nearsightedness, is laser vision correction (LASIK, LASEK, or PRK). Other approaches are being investigated.

In **nearsighted** people, the eyeball is either too long or the cornea has too much curvature. Light focuses on a point in front of the retina; as a result, near objects can be seen clearly, but distant

The Anatomy of Vision Disorders

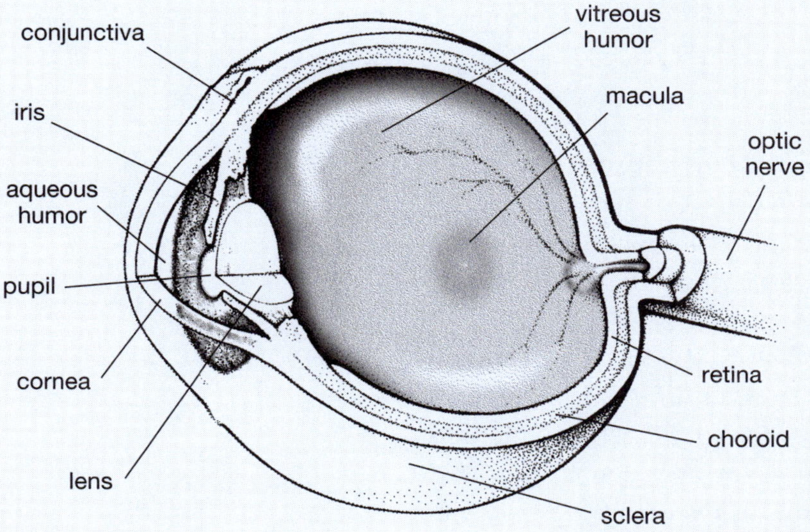

There are 4 leading causes of low vision and blindness in the United States: cataracts, glaucoma, age-related macular degeneration (AMD), and diabetic retinopathy. Each involves a different part of the eye. Cataracts cloud the eye's normally clear lens. Glaucoma, caused by a problem with the drainage of aqueous humor from the eye, damages the optic nerve. Both AMD and diabetic retinopathy affect the sensitive nerve tissue in the retina: AMD destroys the macula—the part of the retina that allows detailed vision—and diabetic retinopathy damages the tiny blood vessels that supply the retina. ■

ones do not come into proper focus. More than 30 million Americans age 40 years and older are nearsighted.

In **farsighted** people, the eyeball is too short or the cornea is too flat, and light focuses on a point behind the retina. Distant objects can be seen clearly, but close ones do not come into proper focus. About 12 million people age 40 years and older in the United States are farsighted.

Astigmatism occurs when the cornea or lens is slightly irregular in shape. This causes light to focus at different points in the eye. The result is blurred or distorted vision. Astigmatism is common in people with nearsightedness.

Presbyopia occurs when the lens begins to lose its ability to accommodate. As we age, the lens gradually becomes thicker and more rigid and is less able to change its shape to bring close objects into focus. Presbyopia affects almost all people over age 45. The primary treatment is reading glasses. Some surgical treatments are currently available, but new procedures are being investigated. If the person is also nearsighted or has astigmatism, prescription bifocals, trifocals, or contact lenses are required.

Cataracts

A cataract is an opacification (cloudiness) of the eye's normally clear crystalline lens. Derived from the Latin word meaning "waterfall," the term cataract arose from the ancient misconception that cataract symptoms were caused by evil liquids that mysteriously flowed into the eye.

Cataracts can occur at any age (in fact, babies can be born with them), but they are most common later in life. About 50% of people age 65–74 and 70% of those age 75 and older have cataracts. In 2004, an estimated 20.5 million Americans over age 40 (approximately 17%) had a cataract. That number is expected to reach 30.1 million by 2020.

Cataract surgery is the most commonly performed surgical procedure in the United States. More than 1.5 million cataract operations are performed each year. However, not all cataracts affect vision significantly or require treatment.

TYPES OF CATARACTS

The lens is made of protein fibers arranged in a specialized way so that the lens is transparent. The lens has 4 distinct layers: At the center is the **nucleus**, which is surrounded by the next layer, the **cortex**. Surrounding the cortex is the **lens epithelium**. The layer at the surface is the **lens capsule**.

Ordinarily, light rays reflected from an object enter the eye through the cornea and lens, which together focus the light onto the retina to produce a sharp image. When a cataract develops, however, light rays are no longer precisely focused. Instead, the rays are scattered before reaching the retina.

The 3 common types of cataracts are defined by where they occur in the lens: **nuclear**, **cortical**, and **posterior subcapsular** (in the rear of the lens capsule). Nuclear cataracts are the most common, and their incidence increases with age and smoking. Cortical cataracts also become more common with age and are related to lifetime exposure to ultraviolet light. Posterior subcapsular cataracts are most likely to occur in younger people and are often the result of prolonged use of corticosteroids (such as prednisone), inflammation, trauma, or diabetes. A person may have more than one type of cataract in the same eye.

The extent of vision damage and how quickly vision becomes impaired depend not only on the size and density of the cataract, but also on its location in the lens. For example, a cataract on the outside edge of the cortex has little effect on vision because it doesn't interfere with the passage of light through the center of the lens, while a dense nuclear cataract causes severe blurring of vision.

CAUSES OF CATARACTS

The cause of most cataracts is unknown, but at least 2 factors associated with aging contribute to cataract development. First, clumping of proteins in the lens leads to scattering of light and a decrease in the transparency of the lens. Second, the breakdown of lens proteins leads to the accumulation of a yellow-brown pigment that clouds the lens.

Researchers have found certain chemical changes in the eyes of people with cataracts. These changes include a reduced uptake of oxygen by the lens and a rise in the water content of the lens, which is later followed by dehydration. When cataracts form, levels of calcium and sodium in the lens increase, and levels of potassium, vitamin C, and protein decrease. In addition, lenses with cataracts appear to be deficient in the antioxidant glutathione. However, studies on the use of medications or vitamins to alter the levels of these substances in the lens have not produced promising results.

Currently, there is no effective drug therapy to prevent cataracts from forming. But cigarette smoking, certain drugs, eye injuries, sunlight, diabetes, and even obesity can increase the risk of cataracts.

Cigarette Smoking

Cigarette smoking appears to raise the risk of developing a cataract. Studies of male physicians and female nurses found an increased incidence of nuclear and posterior subcapsular cataracts in those who smoked the most. Smoking at least 20 cigarettes a day more than doubled the risk of these types of cataracts in men. In women, smoking at least 35 cigarettes a day raised the risk by about 50%. It is not clear why cigarette smoking has an adverse effect on the lens. One possibility is that smoking may reduce blood levels of nutrients required for lens maintenance.

NEW RESEARCH

Sebaceous Carcinoma of the Eyelids

Sebaceous carcinoma is a malignant cancer that generally arises in the sebaceous glands of the eyelids. It usually occurs on the upper eyelid and can metastasize to nearby lymph nodes and distant organs.

In the largest review of cases published to date, researchers evaluated 60 cases of sebaceous carcinoma treated over a 20-year period in Philadelphia.

The patients' median age was 72 years; 73% were women and 27% men. In 24 of the patients, the initial sign of the cancer was a distinct nodule or mass and diffuse eyelid thickening, usually with inflammatory signs.

Sebaceous carcinoma often masquerades as other benign and malignant lesions, often resulting in delayed diagnosis. That was true in this study, with a mean duration of signs and symptoms of 23 months before correct diagnosis.

As of the last follow-up, 53 of the 60 patients were alive and well, and 1 was alive with metastasis. Six had died, 3 of metastasis and the other 3 of other causes. It is hoped that, with more modern treatments available, this type of eyelid cancer will be diagnosed and treated sooner.

OPHTHALMOLOGY
Volume 111, page 2151
December 2004

Corticosteroids

Long-term use of corticosteroids, especially at high doses, is the most common drug-related cause of cataracts. In a study of individuals taking oral prednisone for 1–4 years, cataracts developed in 11% of those taking less than 10 mg a day, in 30% of those taking 10–15 mg a day, and in 80% of those taking more than 15 mg a day. Short-term use of oral corticosteroids is unlikely to lead to cataracts.

Inhaled corticosteroids also can raise the risk of cataracts. In one study, people who had used inhaled corticosteroids had a 50% greater occurrence of nuclear cataracts and a 90% greater occurrence of posterior subcapsular cataracts than those who had not used inhaled corticosteroids. In another study, people using inhaled corticosteroids for more than 3 years were 3 times more likely to need cataract surgery than those who did not use these medications. In addition, the larger the dose of the inhaled corticosteroid, the greater the likelihood of cataract surgery. These results may cause concern for people with asthma, who often rely on inhaled corticosteroids to treat their condition. However, the benefits of inhaled corticosteroids for asthma outweigh the long-term risk of cataracts, which are treatable.

Cataracts can also develop from applying topical corticosteroids to the eyelids or using corticosteroid-containing eyedrops (though the more common side effect is elevated intraocular pressure, which can lead to glaucoma). To reduce the chance of these adverse effects, topical corticosteroids and corticosteroid-containing eyedrops should be used only under the supervision of an ophthalmologist.

Eye Injuries

Blunt trauma to the eye or damage to the eye from certain chemicals can cause clouding of the lens, either immediately or later on. Rapid formation of cataracts commonly occurs after a penetrating eye injury.

Sunlight and Ionizing Radiation

Population studies have shown that prolonged exposure to the ultraviolet (UV) radiation in sunlight more than doubles the risk of cortical cataracts. In one study, the risk of developing cortical cataracts was 2 times greater in people with the highest levels of sunlight exposure than in those with the lowest exposure levels. In addition, the more sunlight exposure, the higher the risk of cortical cataracts. However, the study found that nuclear cataracts were not

NEW RESEARCH

Eye Injuries in the United States

Falls and foreign bodies are the most common causes of eye injuries in the United States.

In a comprehensive survey of eye injuries that took place during 2001, researchers tracked nearly 2 million eye injuries requiring treatment, the equivalent of 6.98 injuries per every 1,000 people.

The pattern of injury rates for males and females was similar across age groups, although males had consistently higher rates. The researchers note that this gender difference virtually disappeared in the oldest age groups.

For white men and women, the injury rates were highest for those in their 20s and 50s. The injury rate among black men was highest in their 30s, 40s, and 70s; the rate among black women was highest in their 30s, 50s, and 70s.

Superficial injuries were most common, followed by foreign body injuries and then being struck against or by an object. The rate for eye injuries caused by falls was higher among women, while rates for injuries related to machinery and objects that cut or pierce the eye were higher among men. Foreign body injuries were more common among older age groups.

ARCHIVES OF OPHTHALMOLOGY
Volume 123, page 910
July 2005

Genetics Update

The role of heredity in eye disease

The Conundrum of Research

One day, research in molecular genetics will open many doors in terms of the diagnosis and treatment of eye diseases such as glaucoma and age-related macular degeneration. Overall, however, we're not there yet.

Challenges include the following:

• **We have a gene, but no test.** For many years, ophthalmologists have known that AMD tends to run in certain families. The strongest evidence yet of a genetic component to the disease came last spring, when 4 independent teams of researchers came up with the same finding: People who inherit a particular form of one gene have a 3–7-fold greater risk of developing AMD.

The researchers implicated one of several variants of the gene that encodes a protein called complement factor H (CFH). Normally, CFH helps regulate inflammation in part of the immune system that attacks diseased and damaged cells. This version of the gene may fail to put the brakes on inflammatory proteins such as C-reactive protein. And that possibility is an intriguing one, as C-reactive protein, which is a systemic marker of inflammation in the body, plays a role in a number of diseases, including AMD and cardiovascular disease (see feature on page 32). All told, this variant of the CFH gene might be responsible for 43–50% of AMD risk, the reports suggested.

However, while these studies confirm that there is a strong genetic component to AMD, and they give researchers a new area to focus on, ophthalmologists and their patients—particularly those with a family history of AMD—are a long way from having a practical blood test to screen for the disease. Eventually, when a blood test is developed, it's possible that it could be used in conjunction with new imaging technologies to detect the earliest signs of AMD.

One additional caveat: As with many diseases, environmental factors still play a significant role in AMD. In a separate study of 840 male twins published last year, genetic factors were estimated to explain 46–71% of the variation in the severity of the disease, with environmental factors such as cigarette smoking and obesity accounting for the remaining 29–54%.

• **We have tests, but no new treatment.** Screening tests are available for 2 of the genes that cause primary open-angle glaucoma. But many glaucoma specialists are reluctant to order them because they have no gene-specific therapy to offer the average person other than additional "watchful waiting."

The tests target 2 of the genes that cause open-angle glaucoma: myocilin and optineurin. Mutations in myocilin (also called TIGR or GLC1A) cause almost all cases of familial juvenile-onset open-angle glaucoma, and 3–5% of cases that occur in adults. Mutations in optineurin (also called OPTN or GLC1E) cause less than 1% of adult-onset cases of open-angle glaucoma.

But while the myocilin and optineurin tests will indicate whether you do or don't have the gene mutation, they can't predict whether you will go on to develop glaucoma. And again, if the gene variant is detected, that diagnosis won't radically change your life— there is no different or specific treatment to offer you.

The only rationale for testing might come in families with a very strong history of juvenile-onset glaucoma. In those cases, if a child or adolescent with the disease is found to have a mutation in the myocilin gene, it might be appropriate to test other children in the family to see if they have the same mutation. If that proves to be the case, then those children should be rigorously monitored for any early signs of disease development.

When Testing Makes a Difference

In contrast to glaucoma and AMD, the future is here when it comes to retinoblastoma, the most common intraocular cancer of childhood that affects some 300 children a year.

The so-called retinoblastoma gene, Rb1, was among the first cancer-causing genes to be detected. Retinoblastoma can be inherited; it also can occur spontaneously. About 90% of cases are detected in children aged 3 years and younger. While treatment is available with radiation or chemotherapy, recent research has found that children who have been successfully treated for the primary cancer with radiation are at increased risk of developing other, fatal cancers outside of the eye, particularly bone cancer and malignant melanoma.

When one parent is known to carry a defective Rb1 gene, reproductive decisions can be agonizing. But it is now possible to pre-select embryos that don't carry the gene via a procedure known as pre-implantation genetic diagnosis (PGD).

The process uses in vitro fertilization (the so-called "test tube baby" technique). After an egg is successfully fertilized, when the embryo reaches the 8-cell stage, one cell is removed and tested for the Rb1 gene mutation. If the test is negative, the embryo can be implanted in the uterus. The technique doesn't disturb or change anything in the embryo's genetic makeup. And not only does the child not have the gene—and not develop retinoblastoma—but also the child will not pass the disease on to any child that he or she might eventually have.

This application of genetics is a relatively recent advance; to date, at least 2 healthy, Rb1-free children have been born thanks to PGD. ■

linked to sunlight exposure. Ionizing radiation (from x-rays, for example) also can cause cataracts.

Diabetes

People with diabetes are at increased risk for cataracts, particularly the posterior subcapsular type, and they tend to be affected at an earlier age than people who don't have diabetes. Some evidence indicates that the accumulation of sorbitol (a sugar formed from glucose) in the lens promotes cataract formation in people with diabetes.

Obesity

Being overweight may also put you at risk for developing cataracts. Proper weight is often determined using body mass index (BMI), a measure of weight in relation to height. To calculate your BMI, multiply your weight in pounds by 704 and divide that sum by the square of your height in inches. Overweight is defined as a BMI between 25 and 29.9; obesity is defined as a BMI of 30 or greater.

In one study of men between the ages of 40 and 84, those whose BMI was between 22 and 28 had roughly a 50% increase in cataract risk, compared with those whose BMI was less than 22. Having a BMI higher than 28 more than doubled cataract risk. Posterior subcapsular cataracts were most often associated with a high BMI. Other studies have found similar results in women.

Although the reason for the link between obesity and cataracts is unclear, it is thought that maintaining a proper weight may reduce cataract formation by decreasing blood glucose levels or by improving the antioxidant properties of the blood.

SYMPTOMS OF CATARACTS

Cataracts form painlessly. The most common symptom is cloudy or blurry vision. Everything becomes dimmer, as if seen through glasses that need cleaning. Most often, both eyes are affected, though vision is usually worse in one eye than in the other. Other symptoms include glare, halos, poor night vision, a perception that colors are faded or that objects are yellowish, and the need for brighter light when reading. In some cases, double vision occurs. This is caused by the passage of light through a lens that has irregular areas of opacity, which can split the rays of light from a single object and focus them on different parts of the retina. Another symptom of cataracts is the need for frequent changes in eyeglass

Cataracts and Vision

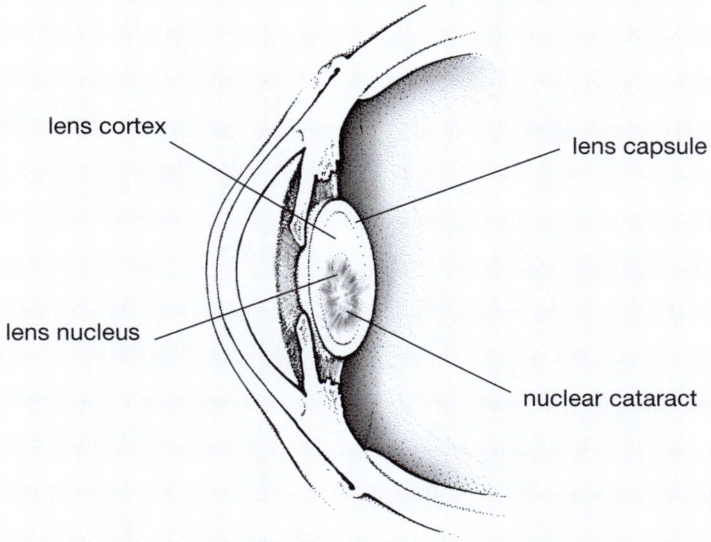

A cataract is a clouding of the lens of the eye that interferes with clear vision. Unlike a healthy, transparent lens, which focuses light rays precisely onto the retina, a lens clouded by a cataract loses its ability to focus light rays. The light that reaches the retina is scattered and diffuse, causing blurry vision.

The amount of vision impairment depends on the size and density of the cataract and where it is located in the lens: the nucleus, cortex, or posterior lens capsule. A cataract in the periphery of the cortex, for example, has little effect on vision because it does not impede the passage of light through the center of the lens. On the other hand, a dense nuclear cataract causes severe blurring, interfering primarily with distant vision (at first). Cataracts that develop in the posterior capsule have a greater effect on near vision and also causes sensitivity to glare. ■

and contact lens prescriptions. These symptoms can develop rapidly (in a matter of months) or almost imperceptibly, over many years.

In the early stages of a nuclear cataract, some people may temporarily have an improvement in vision. For example, a person who previously needed reading glasses for presbyopia is able to read without them. This change, which is referred to as second sight, occurs because the cataract alters the shape of the lens, making it better able to focus on nearby objects. Over time, however, this improvement in vision is lost, and progression of the cataract impairs vision.

Individuals with cortical or posterior subcapsular cataracts often have worse vision in bright light; for example, they may have problems with night driving because of the brightness of oncoming headlights. Bright light causes the pupils to contract and restricts the passage of light to the center of the lens (the part that may be most severely affected by the cataract).

NEW RESEARCH

Lead Exposure and Cataract Risk

Exposure to lead early in life may raise cataract risk later on.

In the Normative Aging Study, a long-running men's aging study, lead emerged as a risk factor for nearly half of the cataracts in men over 60 years of age.

Lead taken into the body is incorporated into bone. Of the 642 men who had their bone lead levels measured, 122 developed cataracts during the follow-up period.

After adjusting for smoking and other risk factors known to contribute to cataract development, those men who had the highest levels of lead in their shin bones were 3 times more likely to have cataracts as were those who had the lowest levels. Overall, the researchers concluded that in the specific population they studied 42% of the cataracts that occurred could be attributed in part to a person's previous lead exposure.

The data suggest that lead exposure is an unrecognized risk for cataract

One positive note: Because leaded gasoline is a thing of the past in the United States and today's young adults and children are less likely to be exposed to lead paint, they might be less likely to develop cataracts than their parents and grandparents.

JOURNAL OF THE AMERICAN MEDICAL ASSOCIATION
Volume 293, page 2750
December 8, 2004

Vision and Alzheimer's Disease

The problem may not be your eyes

Where are those darn car keys? Why can't I remember her name?

Fears of Alzheimer's disease (AD) have us all second-guessing even the most routine of memory lapses. Indeed, impaired memory is one of the classic early signs of the disease.

But in a few people, memory problems aren't the first sign of trouble. Instead, the first sign is problems with vision, or more accurately, problems with visual comprehension. A person may end up in an ophthalmologist's office complaining, "I can't see," or even, "I can see, but I can't read or write." Depth perception may be off, leading to falls and other accidents.

People with these symptoms may have what's known as the visual variant of Alzheimer's disease, or VVAD. While VVAD is relatively uncommon today, it is expected to become more prevalent as the U.S. population ages and more people develop Alzheimer's.

Because the visual comprehension problems come first in VVAD, ahead of those related to memory, people who are affected may consult an ophthalmologist first, thinking that they just need new glasses or even cataract surgery.

Pinning It Down

Whenever a person claims that he or she "can't see," an ophthalmologist begins by assessing the person's visual acuity and visual fields.

While some people with VVAD do show some degree of visual field loss, others have normal eye exams. In a study of 8 patients with VVAD, for instance, only half had any visual field loss. Moreover, the person's visual acuity may be as good as 20/20.

In other words, the problem is not that people with VVAD can't see what's in front of them, it's that their brains aren't accurately processing the information.

In order to screen out VVAD or any other neurologic problem, the ophthalmologist might use one or more of the following tests during the exam:

Clock test. The person will be asked to draw the face of a clock and to draw the clock hands pointing to a specific time, such as 3 p.m. People with VVAD might be unable to draw the clock hands—or they might draw the hands but pointing in the wrong direction. Alternatively, they may be unable to place the numbers on the clock face in the proper sequence. For instance, numbers may be bunched together in one spot on the clock or written out of order, or both.

This simple test is considered a quick, effective initial screening test for VVAD and other forms of dementia. Despite its apparent simplicity, it's actually a complex visual-spatial task: In order to accurately complete it, you must be able to remember where things go in relation to one another and reproduce the correct pattern.

Picture interpretation test. The person will be shown a picture from a book or magazine and asked to describe what's going on in the picture. Someone with VVAD may be able to recognize parts of the scene but may have trouble comprehending the "big picture" and describing the scene in its entirety. For example, if shown an image of a garden in full bloom, the person may be able to identify flowers or trees, but will not be able to explain that the picture is of a garden.

Brain scans. Neuro-ophthalmologists may use magnetic resonance imaging (MRI) and positron emission tomography (PET) scans to help pin down a diagnosis. MRI scans of people with VVAD show some atrophy in the parietal or occipital areas of the brain (the occipital areas interpret vision, while the parietal areas interpret sensory input from the rest of the body and control body movement). PET scans typically show areas where the brain isn't using glucose as expected. Both types of scans may be needed, as the MRI scan may look normal while the PET scan confirms that, in fact, a problem exists.

What's Next?

Once an ophthalmologist suspects VVAD, the individual will be referred to a neurologist for further evaluation and treatment.

While the visual symptoms may be the initial—or in rare cases, the only—sign of Alzheimer's disease, it does appear that most people with VVAD go on to develop the classic symptoms, including impaired memory and personality changes.

It's also important to note that many people with Alzheimer's disease who first experience memory problems typically develop visual problems later on. For instance, they often develop problems with contrast sensitivity or visual attention.

Contrast sensitivity involves the ability to detect different shades of gray. It's an important consideration with nighttime driving, for instance, but it also helps us "read" complex surfaces.

Visual attention has several components: It refers to our ability to detect and identify objects in space, to pay attention to two things at once, and to tune into one type of information while ignoring other less important types of information.

Problems with contrast sensitivity and visual attention play a role in the early stages of Alzheimer's disease, such as problems with driving a car. Later on, they contribute to such well-known problems as being unable to recognize faces or navigate familiar places. As with VVAD, it's important for family members to understand that the person's visual problems are part of the disease and can't be fixed with glasses or surgery. ■

PREVENTING CATARACTS

Since smoking contributes to the risk of developing cataracts, stopping smoking is a vital step in cataract prevention. Studies show that former smokers have a lower risk of cataracts than current smokers, although their risk is not as low as someone who has never smoked. Other benefits of quitting smoking include a reduced risk of cancer, lung disease, and coronary heart disease.

Wearing UV-light-blocking sunglasses and a hat with a wide brim will help reduce eye exposure to UV radiation and may reduce the risk of cataracts. Virtually all sunglasses with tinted plastic lenses provide protection against UV radiation; there is no relationship between the cost of a pair of sunglasses and its UV-blocking ability. The American Academy of Ophthalmology recommends that you wear sunglasses when you are out in the sun for extended periods.

Researchers disagree as to whether certain medications can reduce the risk of cataracts. The results of studies of medications, such as aspirin and hormone replacement therapy, have been contradictory.

Some researchers have speculated that the antioxidant vitamins found in foods or vitamin supplements might help prevent cataracts by protecting against free radicals—unstable oxygen molecules that over time can damage various components of the lens. Antioxidants, which are abundant in fruits and vegetables, include beta-carotene, vitamin C, vitamin E, and selenium. Some studies have found a link between high intakes of antioxidants and a reduced incidence of cataracts, but results from the well-respected Age-Related Eye Disease Study found no such benefit from antioxidant supplements.

TREATING CATARACTS

Surgery is the only way to cure cataracts, but not everyone with cataracts requires surgery. Some people can improve their vision with lifestyle changes.

Lifestyle Measures

Wear sunglasses and a wide-brimmed hat when outdoors to reduce glare. Other options include choosing the appropriate type and amount of indoor lighting, using a magnifying glass, and buying large-print reading materials. Getting a stronger prescription for eyeglasses or contact lenses can sometimes be helpful as well.

NEW RESEARCH

Viagra and Vision Loss

There's more evidence that sildenafil (Viagra) and 2 other drugs in its class may cause permanent vision loss.

Early this year, researchers reported on 7 cases of nonarteritic ischemic optic neuropathy (NAION—decreased blood flow to the optic nerve causing reduced vision) that developed soon after the men took Viagra for erectile dysfunction in doses ranging from 25 mg to 100 mg. Six of the men developed vision loss within the first 24 hours; the seventh was affected within 36 hours after taking the drug.

Their final visual acuity in the affected eye ranged from 20/20 (good vision) to only being able to perceive light. In one person, both eyes were affected.

All of the men had one or more risk factors for heart disease—hypertension, diabetes or high cholesterol levels, which are also known risk factors for NAION.

A follow-up warning from the FDA, issued to physicians in July, 2005, notes that cases of NAION have also been reported in men who took tadalafil (Cialis) or vardenafil (Levitra) for erectile dysfunction. Like Viagra, Cialis and Levitra are phosphodiesterase-5 inhibitors.

The data show that Viagra may trigger NAION in men at high risk for heart disease.

JOURNAL OF NEURO-OPHTHALMOLOGY
Volume 25, page 9
March 2005

Cataract Surgery

Surgery for cataracts involves removing all or part of the lens and replacing it with an intraocular lens implant (IOL). Cataract removal is the most frequently performed surgery in people over age 65 and is considered by many doctors to be the most effective surgical procedure in all of medicine.

If the eye is normal except for the cataract, surgery will improve vision in more than 95% of cases. Because most IOLs are designed to correct nearsightedness or farsightedness, 85% of people who have cataract surgery achieve at least 20/40 vision—good enough to drive a car—1 year after surgery. (People with 20/40 vision are able to see at 20 feet what a person with normal vision can see at 40 feet.) After cataract surgery, however, most people will still need to wear glasses to read small print or do close-up work.

Cataract surgery is remarkably safe. Significant post-surgical complications, such as inflammation, infection, bleeding, swelling, retinal detachment, and glaucoma are rare and occur in only 1–2% of people. People with other eye diseases and serious medical problems are most at risk for complications.

An Overview of Cataract Surgery

Before the 1970s, most surgeons performed cataract surgery with the naked eye or with the aid of loupes—specialized glasses that provide a small amount of magnification. Today, microsurgery is standard and an operating microscope (placed over the eye undergoing surgery) is used that magnifies the eye 4–6 times its normal size.

If you have cataracts in both eyes, the eyes will be operated on at separate times to allow you and your surgeon to assess the outcome of the first surgery. The interval between surgeries gives the first eye time to recover and gives the surgeon a chance to perform the second operation differently if there were complications the first time. Also, if the results with the first eye are good enough, a second operation may not be needed.

Cataract surgery usually takes less than 30 minutes to perform. About 90% of the surgeries are done on an outpatient basis with a local anesthetic, given either by injection or eyedrops. (Local anesthetics render a targeted tissue or part of the body insensitive to pain or sensation. General anesthesia, used only in people who are allergic to local anesthetics or who are extremely anxious, cause complete unconsciousness and relaxation, and prevent pain in the entire body.) Sometimes physicians administer a sedative before the surgery that makes you drowsy and relaxed.

New Intraocular Lenses (IOLs)

Custom-made vision correction

The world of cataract surgery is changing at a blistering pace. A number of new intraocular lenses (IOLs) have recently been approved by the FDA, and others are in the pipeline.

Here are some developments worth watching:

Blocking blue light. Can an IOL that blocks blue-wavelength light help prevent age-related macular degeneration (AMD)? Developers of the AcrySof Natural IOL, which blocks both ultraviolet and blue light, believe that it might do exactly that.

Why bother blocking blue light at all? A few—but not all—observational studies suggest that there may be an association between long-term exposure to blue-wavelength or visible light and AMD. And in the laboratory, recent studies indicate that blue-wavelength light may damage the retina by contributing to the development of free radicals. Theoretically, then, filtering some of the blue light might reduce the formation of these free radicals.

But this doesn't prove that a one-to-one relationship between blue light and AMD exists. Far more research is needed to show whether and how a blue-blocking IOL might affect either the development or progression of AMD. As the IOL's critics point out, controlled photochemical damage in a lab setting is not the same thing as aging of the human retina. Moreover, AMD is a disease with many contributing factors, including genetics.

Another issue that concerns them is that the spectrum of blue light is vital for vision in low light conditions, such as at night or in a dimly lit room. Will the AcrySof Natural IOL's ability to filter blue light interfere with vision in some patients? If this proves to be the case in too many people, it could sink the blue-blocker IOL.

Seeing near to far. The true "Holy Grail" of IOL research is a lens that allows people to see at all distances—near, intermediate, and far. While we're not quite there yet, we get a little closer with the introduction of each new accommodative and multifocal IOL. (Both accommodative and multifocal IOLs provide distance and near vision.)

Last year, the FDA approved the ReZoom and the Restor, both of which are multifocal IOLs. They join the Crystalens, an accommodative IOL, and the Array, a multifocal IOL. All have been shown to reduce a person's overall dependence on glasses or contacts following cataract surgery. However, each type has its pros and cons, making the process of matching the right IOL to the right person an increasingly complex task. For instance, near-sighted people who want to retain their ability to read and do close-up work (such as sewing) won't be happy with the Array or Crystalens, as neither IOL consistently provides optimal reading ability at close distances.

The cost of these new IOLs is too great for many older people with cataracts. But last year, the federal government ruled that Medicare patients who want to have one of the newer IOLs implanted have the option of paying privately for it. Pricing for the Crystalens, ReStor, and ReZoom IOLs ranges from $825–895 —roughly $700 over the standard Medicare reimbursement for a conventional IOL.

IOLs vs. LASIK. If you don't have a cataract or any other eye disease and simply want to get rid of your glasses or contacts, is LASIK the answer? For many people, the answer is "yes." But others—especially those who are severely near- or farsighted—are discouraged from having LASIK, as they are more likely to end up with unsatisfactory results.

One potential solution: phakic IOLs, also known as "implantable contacts." These IOLs are considered best for severely near-sighted people, those who often want LASIK the most, as they literally can't get out of bed and walk across the room without putting on their glasses. They may be a good option for younger people, with the thought that the phakic IOL can tide them over until cataracts form. To date, the Verisyse IOL is the only phakic IOL on the U.S. market; a second one, the Visian lens, is expected to be approved by the FDA.

Accommodative and multifocal IOLs also are being recommended as an alternative to LASIK, especially for people who are far-sighted or have presbyopia (the inability to focus on near objects, which commonly develops in our 40s).

Customized IOLs. Here's a vision from the future: You have an IOL implanted, then your doctor uses a laser to adjust the IOL to account for issues such as near-sightedness or astigmatism. That's the theory behind the Light Adjustable Lens. The light from the laser causes the targeted area of the IOL to swell slightly, which changes its refractive power. The shape can be adjusted several times before the final refraction is "locked in." The IOL is being tested in clinical trials in Mexico and the next step will be European studies.

Another IOL that's still in development and considered promising is the SmartIOL. This is composed of a "smart," flexible polymer that is formed into a rod and inserted through a very small incision. As the rod warms to body temperature, it changes shape and size, expanding and filling the capsule bag completely, just as the natural human lens does. It's considered an accommodative IOL.

Industry observers are keeping close tabs on these IOLs, as both could revolutionize the world of cataract surgery. However, it will be several years before either is available in the United States. ■

Presurgical Tests

Before your surgery, the ophthalmologist will ask about your medical history, which includes past and current medical conditions, current medications, and allergies. An A-scan ultrasonogram, a test that uses sound waves, or a similar test that uses a laser to measure the length of the eyeball, is routinely performed. The eyeball length is used to determine the appropriate focusing power of the IOL that you will receive. If the surgeon cannot see the retina in the back of the eye because the cataract is too opaque, another test called B-scan ultrasonography is used. This test uses reflected sound waves to look at structures in the back of the eye.

Types of Cataract Surgery

Intracapsular surgery. In this approach, the entire lens—the capsule, cortex, and nucleus—is removed. The procedure is rarely performed today but is used in some situations, such as when the lens is partially or completely dislocated.

The surgeon makes an incision at the side of the cornea and then inserts a cryoprobe (a rod with an extremely cold tip) through the incision. When the tip of the probe touches the lens, it adheres to it—as a tongue might stick to a cold metal object in the winter—and the surgeon guides the lens out of the eye as the probe is withdrawn. The incision is closed with multiple fine sutures.

Extracapsular surgery. This type of surgery became popular when surgeons realized that it minimizes trauma to the eye and is associated with fewer postoperative complications than intracapsular surgery. In this approach, the surgeon makes an incision at the side of the cornea and removes the front of the lens capsule, followed by the nucleus and cortex. The back of the lens capsule remains intact and provides support for the lens implant. Most extracapsular surgery is performed using phacoemulsification.

Phacoemulsification. This is the most commonly used technique for cataract surgery. As with the traditional extracapsular procedure, the surgeon makes an incision at the outer edge of the cornea and inserts a needle to cut away the front of the lens capsule. However, instead of using standard surgical tools to remove the cataract, the surgeon then inserts a thin probe. Once activated, the probe emits ultrasonic vibrations that break the cortex and nucleus of the lens into tiny fragments, which are then vacuumed away through a thin tube. At this point, a lens implant can be inserted to replace the missing lens.

The major advantage of phacoemulsification is that its smaller surgical incision helps speed up postoperative healing. Recovery time can be further reduced when phacoemulsification is used in conjunction with a foldable intraocular lens implant, which is inserted and then unfurled inside the eye. When these techniques are combined, the incision can be up to 70% smaller than that with standard extracapsular surgery—so small that it often heals without stitches.

Replacing the Lens

Once the lens is surgically removed, it is usually replaced with an IOL, glasses, or contact lenses to replace the function of the lens and enable clear vision.

Intraocular lens implants. In most cases, once the first phase of the surgery is over and the cataract has been removed, an IOL will be put into place. The quarter-inch plastic lens implant is typically inserted into the lens capsule behind the iris (posterior chamber IOL). In cases where the lens capsule is absent, a different kind of IOL may be inserted just in front of the iris (anterior chamber IOL). IOLs have been in wide use since 1977, and are considered very safe and the standard of care. More than 100 brands of IOLs are available, and more are being developed.

Not all people who undergo cataract surgery are candidates for an IOL, however. For example, lens implantation may not be possible in people with certain eye diseases. People with severe, recurrent uveitis (inflammation of the iris, ciliary body, or choroid [see Glossary]); people with proliferative diabetic retinopathy (new blood vessel growth onto the back surface of the vitreous humor); and people with rubeosis iridis (new blood vessel growth on the iris, which usually occurs in diabetes) are sometimes not eligible for surgery.

The most common type of lens implant is the **monofocal** (single-focus) lens. Unlike the natural lens of the eye, a monofocal IOL cannot alter its shape to bring objects at different distances into focus. As a result, the surgeon generally selects a lens that will provide good distance vision, and the person wears reading glasses for near vision. Alternatively, the surgeon can correct one eye for distance and the other for near vision (this is called monovision).

The first **multifocal** IOL, which provides both distance and near vision, was approved by the U.S. Food and Drug Administration (FDA) several years ago. Multifocal lenses contain several rings, all with a common center and each of which permits the user to see at

NEW RESEARCH

Wearing Contacts Overnight

Wearing extended-wear contact lenses (those you can wear while sleeping) is less risky than it used to be, but it still isn't a good idea.

Researchers studied patients who used contact lenses and presented to the hospital with corneal infiltrative events (CIEs; bacteria in the cornea) or corneal ulcer. The investigators compared the patients' visual acuity before presenting to the hospital (according to records from their eye doctors) vs. their visual acuity 6 months after they presented to the hospital.

During the study, 118 patients sought treatment at the hospital for CIEs of varying severity. Of the patients with CIEs who used daily wear contacts, those who used hydrogel or silicone hydrogel had the highest incidence of CIEs. Of patients who used extended wear who had CIEs, those using extended-wear hydrogel or silicone hydrogel lenses also had higher rates of CIEs.

The risk of developing CIEs was 8.1 times higher in those who wore extended wear lenses vs. those who used daily wear lenses, and the severity of the CIEs was greatest in those who used extended-wear hydrogel lenses. In other words, there was an overall 8 times higher incidence of CIEs in those who slept with contact lenses in. The good news from the study is that none of the patients had a significant loss of visual acuity as a result of their CIE.

CLINICAL EXPERIMENTAL OPTOMETRY
Volume 88, page 232
July 2005

a different distance. Although these lenses reduce the need for eyeglasses, many people still have to wear glasses for certain tasks. In addition, multifocal IOLs can cause bothersome visual side effects such as glare and halos. Researchers are working on developing multifocal IOLs that have fewer visual side effects.

The newest type of IOL, called an **accommodating** lens, contains a hinge that allows for both distance and near vision. The FDA approved the first of these devices, the Crystalens, in 2003. Although most people do achieve 20/40 vision or better with this implant, the range of vision can vary, and improvements in near vision may decrease over time. Other accommodating IOLs are under development.

Many of the monofocal and all of the multifocal IOLs available today are foldable. These foldable IOLs can be inserted into a smaller surgical opening than that required for other types of implants, reducing the amount of trauma to the eye and thereby speeding recovery.

Once inserted, lens implants require no care of any kind. As with any device, however, complications can occur. The most common complication is glare or reduced vision when the IOL is not aligned with the pupil.

In general, new eyeglasses are not prescribed until about 3 weeks after cataract surgery because the prescription changes as the eye heals. Still, if the eye is otherwise normal, people with IOLs often have functional vision as early as the first day after surgery.

Glasses. Cataract glasses are an alternative to IOLs after surgical removal of the lens, but are seldom used as they are heavy and awkward. The glasses magnify objects by about 25%, causing them to appear closer than they actually are (a somewhat disorienting sensation). Because of the thickness and curvature of the lenses, cataract glasses magnify objects unequally and so have a distorting effect as well. In addition, they tend to limit peripheral vision. When used, cataract glasses are prescribed 4–8 weeks after surgery.

Contact lenses. Like cataract glasses, contact lenses are not routinely used after cataract lens removal surgery. The lenses provide almost normal vision, but their major drawback is that people often have difficulty handling, removing, and cleaning them. The frequent handling of contact lenses may also increase the risk of eye infection. Because the patient must be able to see when the contacts are not in place, a pair of cataract glasses is also necessary. Like the glasses, contact lenses are prescribed 4–8 weeks after surgery.

After Surgery

Most people experience minimal discomfort after cataract surgery; a mild painkiller (such as acetaminophen [Tylenol]) can be taken if needed. Some redness, scratchiness, or discharge from the eye may occur during the first few days after surgery. In addition, it is common to see a few black spots or shapes (called floaters) drifting through your field of vision.

In some cases, you will need to wear a protective patch over your eye for 24 hours after surgery. Glasses must be worn during the day to avoid trauma to the eye, and an eye shield is used at night for several days to a few weeks to prevent accidentally rubbing or poking the eye while asleep. Vision varies widely when the patch is first removed.

After phacoemulsification, many people notice improvement in their vision as soon as the next day. Even so, it generally takes 2–4 weeks for the eye to "settle down" and for vision to stabilize. In most people, vision remains blurred for several days or weeks, and then gradually improves as the eye heals. In some cases of extracapsular surgery, the sutures in the eye alter the shape of the cornea and result in temporary blurring or defective vision. This problem generally goes away on its own, though it may require removal of the sutures—a simple and painless procedure.

In general, vision improves faster in those who receive IOLs than in those with cataract glasses or contact lenses. However, surgery usually changes the corrective prescription for the eye (even in those with lens implants), and you will need new eyeglasses to correct any remaining nearsightedness or farsightedness. You are considered fully recovered when your eye is completely healed and vision has stabilized, at which time you will receive a final corrective prescription.

Possible Complications of Surgery

Though cataract surgery is associated with a low rate of complications, problems may arise, especially in older adults or in those with general health problems, such as diabetes. You should contact your doctor if any of the following symptoms develop during recovery from surgery: unusual eye pain or aching; persistent redness; bleeding; excessive tearing or discharge; sudden vision changes; or many bright flashes of light.

About 1% of people, particularly those who are very nearsighted, may develop retinal detachment after cataract surgery. This is a vision-threatening condition in which the retina becomes separated from the underlying layers of the eye. Disruption of the back of the

NEW RESEARCH

Ocular Syphilis Stages a Comeback

After the number of cases of syphilis began to decline in the 1990s in the United States and the United Kingdom, the incidence of ocular syphilis also began to decline—until recently. Syphilis is back, and that means ocular syphilis has staged its own comeback.

In a report from a clinic in Manchester, England, 6 new cases of syphilitic uveitis were diagnosed in 2004 alone. This followed a 15-fold increase in the incidence of syphilis in the United Kingdom from 1999 to 2004, including 615 cases in the Greater Manchester area.

Of the 6 people affected, 4 had latent disease, 2 had no rash, and 2 were HIV-positive.

Ocular syphilis mimics other types of inflammatory eye infections; in cases of latent disease, it often does not show up until a person is older.

Patients' symptoms included inflammation of the iris, the ciliary body, and the choroid; inflammation of the retina; and inflammation and deterioration of the optic disk.

All patients were successfully treated with antibiotics.

The British researchers urge physicians to consider syphilitic uveitis in all people who have retinitis and/or retinal vasculitis or in any uveitis of uncertain origin.

EYE
[Electronically published ahead of print]
June 3, 2005

lens capsule during or after surgery (such as during follow-up laser treatment for postsurgical clouding of the capsule) can increase the risk. Cystoid macular edema (a specific pattern of swelling of the central retina) is another common eye-related complication of cataract surgery. The swelling can result in visual impairment that is usually temporary. If the swelling does not go down on its own, eye-drops may be prescribed.

About one in 1,000 people develop an infection of the vitreous humor called endophthalmitis after cataract surgery. If you experience an increasingly red eye, blurred vision, and pain, visit your ophthalmologist immediately. Typically, this condition can be treated with antibiotics and removal of some of the vitreous humor. Other complications of cataract surgery, such as significant bleeding inside the eye or large pieces of the cataract falling into the back of the eye, can happen but are rare.

In up to 20% of extracapsular surgeries, the back of the lens capsule subsequently becomes cloudy and causes vision difficulties similar to those of the original cataract. Fortunately, recent advances in lens material and design have substantially reduced the risk of this complication. When cloudiness occurs, laser treatment (see below) is an effective remedy.

Laser Treatment Following Extracapsular Surgery

A YAG (yttrium, aluminum, and garnet) laser is used to correct vision blurred by clouding of the back of the lens capsule that remains after extracapsular surgery. The YAG laser produces a hole in the back of the lens capsule by focusing a burst of energy onto it. The procedure, called a YAG capsulotomy, leads to prompt clearing of vision.

The risk of retinal detachment with YAG capsulotomy is small, affecting approximately 1 in 300 people within 3–4 years of surgery. This risk is increased in younger people and those who are extremely nearsighted. Therefore, just as the initial decision to have cataract surgery is based in part on balancing possible risks and benefits, similar issues are weighed before YAG treatment.

Glaucoma

Glaucoma, the second leading cause of adult blindness in the United States after age-related macular degeneration (AMD), results from intraocular pressure (IOP) that is too high for the optic nerve to tolerate. About 2.2 million Americans age 40 years and over have

Neuroprotection and Glaucoma

Taking the pressure off of your eyes

Physicians have recently confirmed through large clinical studies that lowering intraocular pressure (IOP) is highly beneficial in reducing vision loss in people with glaucoma. Indeed, the lowering of IOP is the only FDA-approved approach for treating the disease. However, newer approaches are being studied to supplement present therapy in order to reduce the progressive loss of vision in glaucoma even further.

Despite the achievement of the individual target IOP by medical eyedrop treatment, some residual progressive visual field loss can occur. While the present treatments are sufficient to keep most patients from becoming blind in their lifetime, new investigations are being conducted in laboratories to optimize protection.

Researchers are investigating a number of ways to intervene in this process. Overall, their area of research is known as neuroprotection—protecting the retinal ganglion cell from damage.

Retinal ganglion cells are responsible for visual signaling from the eye to target areas in the brain, and their death is the hallmark of glaucoma. The hope of neuroprotection research is that this retinal ganglion cell loss can be slowed, or even stopped altogether.

Leading Contenders

A number of neuroprotection strategies are under investigation. Some use drugs originally developed for other conditions, such as multiple sclerosis. Some of the most promising are as follows:

Memantine (Namenda). This drug is FDA-approved for treating Alzheimer's disease. It is taken orally and appears to protect brain cells from the damaging effects of high levels of glutamate, an amino acid.

Glutamate binds to the NMDA (N-methyl-D-aspartate) receptor on cells, causing a channel to open and sodium and calcium to enter the cells. When glutamate levels are too high, the NMDA receptors are overstimulated, and too much calcium enters the cells, damaging and eventually killing them. Memantine prevents this destructive cascade by binding to the NMDA receptor and preventing too much glutamate from attaching to the cells.

It is suspected that excess glutamate plays a role in glaucoma damage, although the evidence is controversial. Retinal ganglion cells are very sensitive to the toxic effects of too much glutamate, and some animal studies have shown that memantine can protect the retinal ganglion cells from injury.

A large study of memantine in more than 2,000 people with glaucoma is currently under way; the study is expected to end next year.

Brimonidine (Alphagan). This medication is currently used in eye drop form to treat glaucoma by lowering IOP. In animal studies, oral and injected forms of bromonidine show promise as having a protective effect on the optic nerves and the retinal ganglion cells.

In people, brimonidine is being tested and compared with another glaucoma drug, timolol (Timoptic) in 190 people with normal-tension glaucoma (people with IOP readings in the normal range whose glaucoma is worsening). The goal of the study is to see whether there is any difference between the two drugs in terms of visual field stability or deterioration.

It is important to note that the use of brimonidine eyedrops as a neuroprotectant has no definitive evidence in humans.

Glatiramer (Copaxone). This drug, normally used to treat multiple sclerosis, may protect the optic nerve by triggering a mild autoimmune response. Researchers theorize that the autoimmune response is one way the body protects itself from injury to nerve cells. By using glatiramer, researchers hope to boost the autoimmune response to the initial damage and prevent any additional damage. This is a twist on the idea of vaccination. In this case, while the drug is unlikely to prevent glaucoma from occurring in the first place, it may help slow the rate of progression.

To date, some laboratory studies have found that the drug protects retinal ganglion cells in rats, while other studies have not confirmed this finding. It has yet to be evaluated in people with glaucoma.

Looking Ahead

In addition to developing neuroprotective drugs, researchers are looking at ways to repair retinal ganglion cells and re-establish the axons that connect them to the central nervous system. Stem cell research and gene therapy to promote neuro-regeneration (stimulating repair in damaged cells) are two possible approaches.

However, neuro-regeneration—if it's possible—will take many more years to come to fruition than neuroprotection, researchers say. That's because, in part, it's easier to protect existing retinal ganglion cells than it is to replace nerves that have died.

And no matter which neuroprotective drug for glaucoma makes it to market first, it's unlikely that pressure-lowering tactics will be completely abandoned. IOP will still need to be kept under control, given its role in the disease. Thus, it's possible that people with glaucoma may start with IOP-lowering drops and then add neuroprotective drugs to the mix. ■

glaucoma. (Because the condition does not cause symptoms in its early stages, half of those affected are unaware that they have the disease.) Another 5–10 million people are at increased risk for the disorder.

The risk of glaucoma varies with race and age. The condition is more common in blacks and Hispanics than in whites, and it occurs more frequently with increasing age. In one study, the prevalence of glaucoma was about 1% in people age 40–49 years; in those over age 70, it reached 10% in whites and 20% in blacks.

The two main forms of glaucoma are:

- Open-angle, which accounts for 90% of all glaucoma cases in the United States, progresses slowly, and produces no obvious symptoms until its late stages. It is equally common in men and women.
- Closed-angle glaucoma, which accounts for most of the remaining 10% of glaucoma cases and occurs more often in people of Chinese descent and some other Asian groups. Women are at greater risk than men.

Both types of glaucoma can lead to blindness by damaging the optic nerve. People with normal IOP can also suffer damage to the optic nerve—in fact, up to 50% of people with glaucoma do not have elevated IOP levels. Susceptibility to IOP varies from person to person, and risk factors other than IOP play a role in the development of glaucoma. Early detection and treatment of elevated IOP levels can help prevent optic nerve damage.

CAUSES OF GLAUCOMA

Each day, the eye produces about one teaspoon of aqueous humor—a clear fluid that provides nutrients to, and carries waste products away from, the lens and cornea. (In other parts of the body, the blood carries out these functions, but the lens and cornea have no blood supply.) The aqueous humor is produced by the ciliary body, which surrounds the lens. Aqueous humor flows from behind the iris, through the pupil, and into the front chamber of the eye; it then drains from the eye through a spongy network of connective tissue called the trabecular meshwork, where it ultimately enters the bloodstream. An alternate drainage system, the uveoscleral pathway, is located behind the trabecular meshwork. Ordinarily, fluid production and drainage are in balance, and IOP remains between 12 mm Hg (millimeters of mercury, the same units of measurement used for blood pressure) and 22 mm Hg.

General Causes of Glaucoma

Thin corneas. In some people, a normal level of IOP does not exclude optic nerve damage. Thinner-than-normal corneas can make IOP measurements appear to be lower than they actually are. Thin corneas may therefore be a risk factor for glaucoma. The American Academy of Ophthalmology now recommends that people with other risk factors for glaucoma (for example, advanced age, elevated IOP, and black ancestry) have their corneal thickness measured. (See the "New Research" column to the right.)

Optineurin. Defects in the gene that directs the production of another protein found in the trabecular network and retina of the eye, optineurin, have also been associated with glaucoma. But the role of optineurin is not well understood.

Causes of Open-Angle Glaucoma

Blockage. In people with open-angle glaucoma who have higher-than-normal IOP levels, ophthalmologists suspect that a partial blockage of the trabecular meshwork traps the aqueous humor. Exactly how this happens is unclear. As more aqueous humor is produced than is removed, the blockage causes IOP to rise. Initially, IOP does not rise high enough to cause discomfort or any easily perceived changes in vision, but when it remains elevated or continues to rise, fibers in the optic nerve are compressed and eventually die, leading to a gradual loss of vision over several years.

Heredity. Your genetic makeup may also play a role in glaucoma risk. Genetic defects that cause glaucoma have been identified in what's called the chromosome-1 open-angle glaucoma gene (GLC1A), which directs the production of myocilin, a protein found in trabecular meshwork cells. Defective forms of myocilin are thought to block proper drainage of aqueous humor.

Medications. Inhaled and nasally administered drugs that contain corticosteroids, commonly used to treat asthma and allergies, appear to raise the risk of elevated IOP and open-angle glaucoma, possibly by interfering with the drainage of aqueous humor. Oral corticosteroids may have the same effect. If you must use corticosteroids (for conditions such as asthma, arthritis, sinusitis, or chronic bronchitis) you should have your IOP and vision monitored regularly.

Causes of Closed-Angle Glaucoma

Closed-angle glaucoma results when aqueous humor is blocked at the pupil, leading to a bowing forward of the iris that stops aqueous humor from reaching the trabecular meshwork. The blockage

NEW RESEARCH

Corneal Thickness: More than One Measurement is Needed

In glaucoma, the relationship between central corneal thickness and intraocular pressure has come under increased scrutiny, with a major study suggesting a link between central corneal thickness (CCT) and the risk of developing primary open-angle glaucoma.

Thus, if CCT is related to intraocular pressure, it's essential to obtain an accurate CCT measurement. But for that to occur, more than one CCT reading may be needed.

In a study of 51 people with glaucoma, researchers used handheld pachymeters (an instrument that measures corneal thickness) to measure CCT during 2 consecutive clinic visits. The readings not only showed a clear fluctuation over a 3-month period but also demonstrated a systemic bias toward increased corneal thickness being recorded at the second reading.

While CCT readings should be part of the routine assessment of patients, the researchers say, they urge caution, noting that physicians must be sure that their CCT readings are consistent before they make a diagnosis and recommend a treatment plan.

OPHTHALMOLOGY
Volume 112, page 225
February 2005

causes a sudden increase in IOP that can lead to severe, permanent vision damage within just 1–2 days if not treated immediately.

SYMPTOMS OF GLAUCOMA

Open-angle glaucoma generally affects both eyes, although IOP levels and the extent of damage to the optic nerve often differ between eyes. Because of the way the optic nerve is structured, the first nerve fibers damaged are those used for peripheral vision. People with advanced open-angle glaucoma can have 20/20 vision when looking straight ahead but may have blind spots (called scotomas) for images located outside the center of the visual field. The damage is often not detectable on visual field tests (perimetry tests) until as much as 40% of the optic nerve fibers are destroyed. Eventually, the fibers needed for central vision may be lost as well.

Unlike the open-angle form, closed-angle glaucoma sometimes occurs as acute attacks that strike when IOP rises rapidly to a dangerous level. Signs of an attack include severe pain in the eye, nausea and vomiting, blurred vision, and rainbow-colored halos around lights. Attacks typically do not occur in both eyes at once, but after an initial attack there is a 40–80% chance that a similar attack will occur in the other eye within the next 5–10 years if no treatment is provided.

PREVENTING GLAUCOMA

The only methods of preventing glaucoma involve drugs or surgery. For open-angle glaucoma, a 2002 study of more than 1,600 people with elevated IOP and no other signs of glaucoma suggested that IOP-lowering eyedrops delay the development of glaucoma. In the study, 4% of those who took IOP-lowering medication developed glaucoma over a 5-year period, compared with 10% of those who did not take these medications.

For closed-angle glaucoma, making a hole in the iris with a laser can be preventive, although the decision to perform this treatment depends upon a variety of factors.

DIAGNOSING GLAUCOMA

An eye examination for glaucoma involves measuring IOP, viewing the optic nerve, and testing the visual fields. In general, white people should be examined for glaucoma every 2 years after age 50, and black people every 2 years after age 40; optic nerve damage is uncommon before age 50 in whites but can occur up to 10 years earlier in blacks. If you have cardiovascular disease or are severely nearsighted, you may need to begin examinations at a younger age and have more frequent exams because of your increased risk of nerve damage from glaucoma.

IOP measurements alone are no longer used to diagnose glaucoma because some people with elevated IOP do not develop optic nerve damage, while others develop glaucoma despite having a normal IOP reading. A high IOP raises the suspicion of glaucoma, but other tests are required to make a diagnosis.

Tests for Glaucoma

Ophthalmologists use 3 types of tests to screen for and diagnose glaucoma and to monitor progress during treatment:

Tonometry. This test measures IOP by assessing the amount of force needed to flatten a small area of the cornea. The most effective way to do this is with what's known as applanation tonometry. In this test, the eye is numbed with anesthetic eyedrops. Then, slight pressure is applied to the cornea with a small instrument (a tonometer) while the doctor looks through a table-mounted microscope called a slit lamp. A handheld tonometry device (Tono-Pen) is sometimes used for testing as well and is relatively accurate. Tonometry is painless and poses virtually no risk to the cornea.

Air-puff tonometry, in which IOP is measured with a quick puff of warm air, is being re-evaluated for its accuracy as a diagnostic tool. Anesthetic eyedrops are not needed for this procedure because the air-puff tonometer does not touch the eye.

Ophthalmoscopy. This test is used to inspect the optic nerve, both when making the initial diagnosis of glaucoma and when examining the nerve during treatment. To perform ophthalmoscopy, the doctor dilates the pupils with eyedrops, then uses an ophthalmoscope—a special instrument with a small light on the end of it—to magnify and examine the optic nerve. A slit lamp may also be used, as this specialized microscope provides a 3-dimensional view of the nerve. Signs of a damaged optic nerve include "cupping" in its center and a loss of its normal pink color. A number of other imaging techniques, such as laser-based image formation, are used to supplement ophthalmoscopy when confirming a diagnosis of glaucoma.

Perimetry. As with ophthalmoscopy, perimetry is used to help diagnose glaucoma and monitor progression of the disease during treatment. The patient wears a patch over one eye and looks

NEW RESEARCH

When People Don't Take Their Glaucoma Medications

Noncompliance among glaucoma patients is common, but whether this leads to an insufficient reduction in intraocular pressure and progression of visual field loss, and subsequent risks and costs, is unclear.

In a large review of 29 previously published international glaucoma studies, researchers found that many glaucoma patients fail to comply with their prescribed treatment regimen, with the reported proportion of noncompliance ranging from 5–80%.

Even so, it was not possible for the researchers to determine the full impact of this noncompliance on clinical outcome, especially the potential progression of visual field loss.

In their review, the researchers found that men appeared to be less likely to comply than women. They also suggest that patient education may play a role in supporting compliance—the more people know about their disease, the more likely they are to comply —and that treatment regimens that simplify the number of medications and/or the number of drops per day also may support compliance.

OPHTHALMOLOGY
Volume 112, page 953
June 2005

Glaucoma Drugs 2006

Drug Type	Generic Name	Brand Name
Beta-blockers	betaxolol carteolol levobunolol metipranolol timolol	Betoptic-S Ocupress Betagan OptiPranolol Betinol Timoptic Ocumeter Timoptic-XE Ocumeter
Adrenergic agonists	apraclonidine brimonidine dipivefrin epinephrine	Iopidine Alphagan-P Propine Epifrin
Miotics	carbachol echothiophate pilocarpine	Isopto Carbachol Phospholine Iodide Isopto Carpine Pilocar Pilopine HS Piloptic
Carbonic anhydrase inhibitors	acetazolamide brinzolamide dorzolamide methazolamide	Diamox Azopt Trusopt Ocumeter Neptazone
Topical prostaglandins	bimatoprost latanoprost travoprost	Lumigan Xalatan Travatan
Combination product	dorzolamine-timolol	Cosopt

straight ahead at a bowl-shaped white area, while a computer provides lights at various locations around the bowl. The patient indicates each time he or she sees a light. By documenting the lights the patient can see, perimetry provides a "map" of the visual fields. The type of vision loss associated with glaucoma is relatively specific, and perimetry can detect the visual-field defects that are typical of glaucoma. The test takes about 4 minutes to perform in each eye.

Quicker methods of perimetry that take only 2 minutes per eye are now being used. Among the most promising is frequency doubling technology which measures damage to the type of cells in the retina—ganglion cells—that appear to be more susceptible to damage by glaucoma than the optic nerve. Other newer perimetry methods include the use of colored test lights (blue targets on a yellow background).

How They Work	Comments
These eyedrops decrease the production of aqueous humor.	Lowered pulse rate, low blood pressure, asthma, fainting, drowsiness, confusion, depression, and dry eyes may occur in some people. Beta-blockers usually should not be used by people who have severe lung or heart ailments.
These eyedrops decrease aqueous humor production and increase its drainage.	Associated with the highest rate of allergic reactions. People may also experience red eyes, pain, headaches, eye irritation, high blood pressure, or rapid heart rate. The drops may stain contact lenses (except dipivefrin). Use with caution in people with heart ailments or high blood pressure.
These eyedrops or ointment (Pilocarpine HS) increase drainage of aqueous humor through the trabecular meshwork by constricting the pupil.	People may experience dim vision (especially at night) or increased nearsightedness. Echothiophate may cause cataracts; in general, it is used only when cataracts have been removed.
These oral drugs (acetazolamide and methazolamide) and eyedrops (brinzolamide and dorzolamide) decrease the production of aqueous humor.	Up to 50% of people taking oral carbonic anhydrase inhibitors have side effects, including tingling of the hands and feet, stomach upset, depression, kidney stones, and, more rarely, anemia; thus, these drugs are used only when absolutely necessary to avoid surgery and preserve eyesight. Brinzolamide and dorzolamide eyedrops do not have such side effects.
These eyedrops increase the drainage of aqueous humor from the eye.	A change in eye color is the most noticeable side effect, with about 3% of people experiencing an increase in brown pigmentation. Other side effects include stinging, burning, redness, and foreign body sensation.
See carbonic anhydrase inhibitors and beta-blockers above.	See carbonic anhydrase inhibitors and beta-blockers above.

If you have a high IOP, additional tests will be run. The final diagnosis is made if your doctor finds evidence of optic nerve damage typical of glaucoma or identifies defects characteristic of glaucoma in the visual fields. To distinguish between open-angle and closed-angle glaucoma, the ophthalmologist will examine the front part of the eye to check the angle where the iris meets the cornea.

TREATING GLAUCOMA

Most forms of glaucoma are chronic conditions that cannot be cured. Open-angle glaucoma can often be treated safely and effectively with medication or surgery, but lifelong use of medication is almost always necessary. Decisions on when to start treatment are based on the amount of optic nerve damage and visual field loss, as

Consider Drug Side Effects

Could your medications be causing vision problems?

Vision problems can be an unwanted side effect of many different medications. Most drugs will cause only temporary visual disturbances, such as blurred or double vision, dry eyes, excessive tearing, puffy eyelids, sensitivity to light, seeing a yellow or blue tinge, or a change in eye color. These disappear with time or once the medication is discontinued. However, long-term use of certain medications may result in more serious vision problems.

Always consider drug side effects when visual symptoms develop, and be sure to tell your ophthalmologist about all medications you are taking. Regular use of any drug associated with serious vision disorders merits periodic monitoring of the eyes.

Listed below are some of the most common drugs associated with vision problems.

• Antiarrhythmia drugs, such as amiodarone (Cordarone) and digoxin (Lanoxin), are used to treat abnormal heart rhythms and may cause visual disturbances such as blurred vision, yellow vision, or blue-green halos around objects.

• Antimalarial drugs, such as chloroquine (Aralen) and hydroxychloroquine (Plaquenil), are used not only for malaria, but also for rheumatoid arthritis and lupus. They may cause visual disturbances such as blurred vision, and prolonged therapy may lead to irreversible retinopathy.

• Corticosteroids such as prednisone (Deltasone and other brands) may lead to glaucoma or cataracts. Oral treatments (commonly used for arthritis) are linked to cataracts, while the inhaled versions used to treat asthma are associated with both cataracts and glaucoma.

• Erectile dysfunction drugs, like sildenafil (Viagra), tadalafil (Cialis), and vardenafil (Levitra), can temporarily cause objects to have a blue tinge to them, blurred vision, and sensitivity to light.

• Phenothiazines, like chlorpromazine (Thorazine) and thioridazine (Mellaril), are used to treat schizophrenia. These drugs may lead to blurred vision, changes in color vision, and difficulty seeing at night.

• Tamoxifen (Nolvadex), which is used to reduce the risk of breast cancer recurrences, may lead to blurred vision, changes to the retina and cornea, and cataracts. ■

well as risk factors such as elevated IOP, increasing age, and black or ethnic background.

Acute closed-angle glaucoma is a medical emergency. If you have symptoms of closed-angle glaucoma (severe pain in the eye, nausea and vomiting, blurred vision, and rainbow-colored halos around lights), contact your ophthalmologist immediately.

The overall aim in treating glaucoma—either open-angle or closed-angle—is to prevent damage to the optic nerve by lowering IOP and maintaining it at a level that is unlikely to cause further nerve damage. An appropriate and typical target is to lower IOP by 25% below the level noted when you are diagnosed, although the target is even lower in people with extremely high IOP levels (above 35 mm Hg). Once the target IOP is achieved, you will be monitored to make sure that damage to the optic nerve is not progressing. If there is progressive damage at the target IOP, a lower target will be set. Unfortunately, treatment cannot reverse optic nerve damage once it has occurred and cannot improve vision.

Choosing a treatment for glaucoma involves weighing the health benefits and risks of each option, while trying to minimize overall inconvenience and financial costs. Medication and surgery are both first-line treatments for glaucoma, and each has its own set of complications and possible side effects. In some cases, medication does not stop the progression of optic nerve damage or visual field loss, possibly because the doctor has selected a target IOP that is not low enough, or because the target IOP is not reached (if a person does not take the medication as prescribed, for example). Surgical complications, such as the development of cataracts, occur in only a small number of people, and the risk is lower with laser trabecular surgery than with traditional filtration surgery (see the "Surgery" section on page 30).

Medication

If you have glaucoma, it is essential that you regularly visit your ophthalmologist to have your IOP, visual fields, treatment side effects, and the appearance of the optic nerve monitored. Visits may be as frequent as daily or weekly when treatment first begins and in people with severe optic nerve damage or extremely high IOP levels. Visits may only be needed every 3–6 months in people with stable IOP levels and minimal optic nerve damage.

It is also essential to follow your medication regimen as prescribed by your doctor. Some people have trouble with this, either because they take a large number of other prescription medications, or because they have to take glaucoma medication more than twice a day. In addition, the cost or side effects of glaucoma medication may be difficult to deal with. If any of these factors are affecting your ability to follow your treatment regimen, ask your doctor if any changes can be made to your regimen.

At present, eye doctors treat glaucoma mostly with eyedrops, although oral drugs are occasionally given.

Eyedrops. Eyedrops are the most common medication for glaucoma. In general, they are applied 1–4 times a day at regular intervals. Drops can cause local side effects, such as burning, stinging, tearing, itching, or redness in the eye. They can also cause systemic (affecting the whole body) side effects because some of the drug in the drops is absorbed into the body. However, systemic effects are less of an issue with eyedrops than with oral medications. One example of a common systemic side effect is that beta-blocker eyedrops can lower blood pressure in addition to lowering IOP.

Systemic side effects can be minimized by carefully following instructions for using the eyedrops, including placing a finger on the inside corner of the eye for 2–3 minutes to prevent the eyedrops from entering the nasal ducts.

Five types of eyedrops are currently used (see "Glaucoma Drugs

2006" on page 24 for more information).

Beta-blockers. These drugs lower IOP by reducing the production of aqueous humor. The most commonly used beta-blocker is timolol (Timoptic). Other beta-blockers, such as betaxolol (Betoptic), carteolol (Ocupress), and levobunolol (Betagan) are just as effective. Systemic side effects of beta-blockers include slowed heart rate, reduced blood pressure, reduced libido, anxiety, nausea, vomiting, and breathing difficulties.

Topical prostaglandins. The topical prostaglandins bimatoprost (Lumigan), latanoprost (Xalatan), and travoprost (Travatan) reduce IOP by improving drainage of aqueous humor. These medications appear to be at least as effective as the beta-blocker timolol and are associated with fewer side effects. Consequently, topical prostaglandins are now the most frequently used drugs for glaucoma. These medications are also sometimes used in combination with another glaucoma medication to produce greater reductions in IOP. About 3% of people taking topical prostaglandins for 6 months or more experience gradual changes in eye color—from blue or green to brown. Other possible side effects include burning, stinging, and increased eyelash growth.

Carbonic anhydrase inhibitors. Two carbonic anhydrase inhibitors are available as eyedrops: brinzolamide (Azopt) and dorzolamide (Trusopt). These eyedrops lower IOP by decreasing production of aqueous humor. They are used when other glaucoma medications are ineffective. Common side effects include fatigue, stinging in the eyes, and loss of appetite.

Adrenergic agonists. Adrenergic agonists, such as dipivefrin (Propine) and epinephrine (Epifrin), can increase the drainage of aqueous humor but work primarily by decreasing its production. Possible side effects include burning in the eyes, enlarged pupils, and allergic reactions.

Brimonidine (Alphagan) and apraclonidine (Iopidine) are two other adrenergic agonists. The most common side effects of these two drugs include dry mouth and altered taste. Allergic reactions also may occur.

Miotics. Miotics, such as pilocarpine (Isopto Carpine and other brands) and carbachol (Isopto Carbachol) increase the drainage of aqueous humor by improving its flow through the trabecular meshwork. Side effects of these drugs include nearsightedness and reduced night vision. Excessive tearing, eye pain, and allergic reactions may also occur.

Combination medication. A medication containing both dorzo-

NEW RESEARCH

Women Less Likely to Get Glaucoma Treatment Than Men

Women and younger people are much less likely to receive glaucoma treatment than older men.

In a very large study of 35,754 people suspected of having glaucoma, 5,265 diagnosed with glaucoma, and 2,633 with signs of early glaucoma in a single care organization, researchers studied who received treatment with either surgery or medication. What they found was that treatment in people with glaucoma or suspected of having glaucoma was initiated less often in women, especially if they were younger and not followed-up at their doctor's office. Other variables associated with greater likelihood of treatment were having a diagnosis of glaucoma and the region of the country where the patients were treated.

Women were 24% less likely to be treated than men, and younger people of both sexes were far less likely to be treated than older people.

Since the reasons for the disparity in treatment are unclear, the authors note that understanding the sources of variation in treatment will improve treatment for people with glaucoma or suspected of having glaucoma.

OPHTHALMOLOGY
Volume 112, page 1494
September 2005

Exercise and Glaucoma

Staying fit benefits your eyes

If you've just been diagnosed with glaucoma, you undoubtedly want to do everything you can to be as healthy as possible for as long as possible. As part of that, you may wonder whether changes in your overall lifestyle, including changes in the amount or type of exercise you get, may help control the disease.

While the mainstay of glaucoma therapy remains lowering IOP with medication, laser treatment, or surgery, some evidence does suggest that a regular exercise program can help support your medical therapy.

But what kind of exercise is best? Is there anything in particular you should—or shouldn't—do? Here's an overview of what's known.

Beneficial effects. Overall, exercise has been found to lower IOP. Studies also have found that it improves blood flow to the retina and optic nerve.

In one study, jogging for 20 minutes lowered IOP by 1 mm Hg to 8 mm Hg. In another, weight lifting also lead to decreases in IOP, with IOP dropping by 14.5% after the third set of chest presses and 13.2% after the third set of leg presses.

While the jogging and weight training studies were conducted in healthy, athletic people, exercise has also been found to benefit sedentary people with ocular hypertension. For instance, 3 months of moderate exercise for 9 sedentary people suspected of having glaucoma decreased mean IOP by 4.6 mm Hg (20% for these particular patients).

If you aren't already active, there's no need to adopt a hard-core exercise program. Simply going for a walk three or more times a week is all you need.

The catch? The exercise benefit continues only as long as you continue exercising. In the study of the sedentary glaucoma suspects, just 3 weeks of deconditioning undid the beneficial effects.

Caveats to consider. It's important to avoid the Valsalva effect (the technical term for what happens when, after an inhalation, you hold your breath and apply pressure against your epiglottis), as this appears to have a negative impact on IOP. Thus, if you're interested in weight lifting or other forms of resistance exercise, be sure to get proper training on breathing techniques. The same holds true for yoga and Pilates, as people sometimes incorrectly hold their breath either going into or coming out of a pose.

Another concern regarding yoga: It's best to avoid all inverted poses if you have glaucoma. This includes headstand, shoulderstand, and the plow. While few studies have been conducted on yoga and glaucoma, there is some evidence that inverted poses increase IOP, so be sure to discuss alternative poses or modifications with your yoga instructor.

Bottom line. A regular program of moderate exercise will have multiple benefits for your overall health. While its long-term impact on your glaucoma progression is unknown, it is likely to support your current treatment program. If you have any questions about your existing exercise program, or any concerns about starting a new activity, check with your ophthalmologist. ■

lamide and timolol is available (Cosopt). This drug reduces the production of aqueous humor and has proven more effective in lowering IOP than either drug alone. Cosopt is often used with a topical prostaglandin to reduce IOP in people for whom single-drug therapy is not successful.

Oral medications. Acetazolamide (Diamox) and methazolamide (Neptazane), both carbonic anhydrase inhibitors, are the only glaucoma medications that are taken orally. Because of their side effects, they are generally used only when optic nerve damage continues to worsen despite the use of eyedrops at the highest tolerable dose. The drugs initially lower IOP by 20–30% but are associated with significant systemic side effects (such as numbness or tingling in the hands and feet, malaise, and loss of appetite) and occasional serious complications (such as depression, kidney stones, diarrhea, and damage to blood cells). For more information, see the drug chart on page 24.

Surgery

About 10% of people with open-angle glaucoma undergo surgery due to serious side effects from medications, lack of response to drug treatment, the inability to take their medications properly, or medical conditions or allergies that interfere with drug therapy.

While surgery cannot restore lost vision, it can reduce IOP by improving the drainage of aqueous humor. As a result, surgery can dramatically slow the progression of optic nerve damage and vision loss.

The two most common surgical procedures for open-angle glaucoma are:

Laser trabecular surgery. In this procedure, 80–100 tiny laser burns are made in the area of the trabecular meshwork. The procedure increases the drainage of aqueous humor, most likely by stimulating the activity of trabecular cells. The procedure takes about 15 minutes and is performed on an outpatient basis using eyedrops for anesthesia. IOP must be measured one hour after surgery because it may temporarily rise as a result of the treatment. Postoperative complications are minimal and include eye inflammation, blurred vision, and minimal discomfort, usually lasting for about 24 hours.

It takes up to 6 weeks to determine whether the procedure has been effective. IOP-lowering medication is often still required after surgery, but if the procedure reduces IOP considerably, you may be able to lower the dose of your medication. As with many treatments, however, the effect of surgery diminishes with time in some people. About 40% of people need additional medication or some other form of surgery within 5 years.

Filtration surgery. This type of surgery (technically known as trabeculectomy) uses conventional surgical instruments to open a passage through the trabecular meshwork so that aqueous humor can drain into surrounding tissues. The operation takes about 20 minutes, is performed on an outpatient basis under local anesthesia, and is relatively safe and long-lasting. In general, a protective eye patch must be worn for one day after the procedure, and people are advised to avoid driving, bending over, and performing strenuous activity for at least a week. If necessary, the drainage flap created during the surgery can be loosened or tightened later on with a new laser procedure (called suture lysis) or with the use of special adjustable sutures.

After filtration surgery, about 50% of people are able to stop taking their glaucoma medication; 35–40% still need some medication; and 10–15% need additional surgery, such as shunts or cyclodestructive surgery (see below). Filtration surgery carries a risk of infection and bleeding in the eye, and requires a longer recovery period than laser trabecular surgery. In addition, about one third of people develop cataracts within 5 years of filtration surgery. It is not clear whether the surgery itself causes the cataracts or whether they would have occurred anyway, but the cataracts can be surgically removed when necessary.

Researchers are working to improve the effectiveness of filtration surgery. One of the most promising approaches is the use of antimetabolites (substances that block biological processes) such as mitomycin or 5-fluorouracil. Both mitomycin and 5-fluorouracil can be applied as a liquid during surgery; 5-fluorouracil can also be injected under the surface of the eye after surgery. These drugs interfere with normal wound healing so that the openings created by the procedure do not close. Currently, these antimetabolites are used primarily in people who have had unsuccessful filtration surgery and in younger individuals who normally have strong wound-healing abilities.

Shunts. If filtration surgery is unsuccessful, one alternative is to drain excess aqueous humor using a shunt made of plastic tubing. The shunt is implanted into the front chamber of the eye, and the aqueous humor drains onto a plate sewn onto the side of the eye. The tissues surrounding the eye then absorb fluid on the plate. In one study, a shunt called the Baerveldt implant lowered IOP in 72% of people with previously uncontrolled glaucoma.

Cyclodestructive surgery. This form of glaucoma surgery uses a laser to destroy the ciliary body—a part of the eye that surrounds the lens and produces aqueous humor. Recovery time depends on the type and extent of the surgery. The procedure does not require an incision, so people can return to their normal daily activities earlier than after filtration surgery. Cyclodestructive surgery is usually used only when other measures have failed.

Treating Closed-Angle Glaucoma

During an acute attack of closed-angle glaucoma, IOP may be high enough to damage the optic nerve or block one of the blood vessels carrying blood and oxygen to the retina. Unless IOP is lowered immediately, blindness can occur within days.

Preventing Progression of AMD

Take steps to protect your vision

The advanced stages of macular degeneration are estimated to currently affect more than 1.75 million people in the United States. And based on demographic projections, the prevalence of AMD will increase by 50%, reaching nearly 3 million people in less than 20 years.

Most current treatments are limited to the late stage of the disease, when central vision is already under great threat. Thus, the race is on to find effective strategies for earlier intervention (see page 39, "New Drug for AMD") and even prevention.

Preventing AMD

If you're concerned about AMD, what can you do to help yourself while drug research continues?

The following factors are known to play a role in either hastening or delaying AMD progression and thus are good places to begin:

Smoking. This leads the list: There's no question that smoking is the No. 1 environmental risk factor for AMD. Earlier this year, the Age-Related Eye Disease Study (AREDS) confirmed that smoking increases the risk of progression to advanced AMD among people who have the early or intermediate form of the disease. In addition to increasing oxidative stress, smoking may play a role in AMD by impairing choroidal microcirculation in the eye.

Obesity. Obesity's connection to such diseases as hypertension and diabetes is well known. But obesity in general—and abdominal obesity in particular—also appears to increase the risk for progression to advanced AMD.

Obesity leads to increased oxidative stress and inflammation (thought to play a role in AMD), which may increase destruction and decrease delivery of 2 beneficial nutrients in the eye, lutein and zeaxanthin (found predominantly in green leafy vegetables, such as spinach and kale). These 2 nutrients accumulate in the retina and are the main components of the macular pigment. They are known to function as anti-oxidants and as filters of damaging blue light in the UV spectrum. Researchers theorize that they may protect the macula from light-initiated oxidative damage to the retina and retinal pigment epithelium.

Vitamins. The original Age-Related Eye Disease Study (AREDS) from the National Eye Institute formula— 500 mgs of vitamin C, 400 IU of vitamin E, 15 mg of beta-carotene, 80 mg of zinc, and 2 mg of copper in the form of cupric oxide—delayed progression to end-stage AMD by 25% in those with either intermediate or advanced AMD.

The AREDS formula (sold under the name Outvite Preservation) is clearly indicated for high-risk AMD patients. Researchers have estimated that if all of those at high risk for advanced AMD took the recommended vitamins, approximately 300,000 people could avoid significant vision loss over the next 5 years.

Additional Considerations

The following are possible, but not proven, factors that may affect the progression of AMD. Interestingly enough, they also play a role in cardiovascular disease.

Nutrition. On the dietary front, investigators have found that a high intake of saturated fats and trans-fatty acids is associated with a higher risk for AMD and progression of the disease. Saturated fats (found in red meat, butter, and whole-fat dairy foods) and trans-fatty acids (found in many margarines, snack foods, and baked goods) are proven to raise cholesterol levels. In contrast, diets high in omega-3 fatty acids (recommended for heart disease prevention) may protect against AMD. Omega-3s are found predominantly in fatty fish such as salmon, but they are also found in leafy greens, flaxseeds, and flaxseed and canola oils.

IOP in the affected eye is lowered with medication followed by surgery, either with laser (iridotomy) or, rarely, with conventional incisions (iridectomy). In both cases, surgery involves making a tiny hole in the iris to allow a path for the flow of aqueous humor. Surgery is almost always successful, and repeat treatment is rarely necessary.

In addition to protecting the optic nerve in the affected eye, a goal of treatment is to prevent an acute attack in the other eye, which is highly likely. A preventive iridotomy is therefore usually performed in the other eye. In some people, a chronic form of

A small study drawn from the original AREDS study has found that people who eat more foods containing lutein, zeaxanthin, and omega-3 fatty acids have a significantly lower risk of AMD. Those who ate the most fish per week (2 or more servings) had almost a 50% reduction in AMD risk, while those who ate the most foods containing lutein and zeaxanthin had a nearly 40% reduction in risk.

Based on these findings, the next phase of AREDS (known as AREDS II) will evaluate omega-3s, lutein, and zeaxanthin in at-risk people (those who should already be on the original AREDS formulation). The study is expected to begin during the first part of 2006 and to run approximately 7 years.

C-reactive protein (CRP). CRP, a biomarker of inflammation in the body, is considered an independent indicator of increased risk for cardiovascular and peripheral arterial disease. CRP levels appear to rise with chronic illnesses, smoking, obesity, hypertension, and insulin resistance.

Recent research indicates that CRP is also a systemic inflammatory marker of AMD. Last year, researchers reported that CRP levels were significantly higher among individuals with intermediate and advanced stages of AMD. This effect persisted even after the researchers accounted for the effects of smoking and obesity. The risk of AMD was lowest among those with low CRP values and no smoking history. However, the link with CRP isn't proven, and many questions remain about its role.

Cholesterol-lowering drugs. Because cholesterol, which is involved in the pathogenesis of atherosclerosis, is an important constituent of drusen (lipid deposits in the eye that are a sign of early AMD), a number of researchers have pursed the possibility that lipid-lowering drugs could reduce AMD risk.

The class of drugs known as statins are proven to lower cholesterol levels, and more recent studies have shown that they have broader anti-inflammatory effects and lower CRP levels as well. Some studies have suggested that they might also protect against AMD, thanks not only to their cholesterol-lowering properties but also to their ability to improve endothelium dysfunction (endothelial cells line vessels in the heart, blood, and lymph vessels) and decrease oxidative stress and vascular inflammation. However, the evidence from AMD studies is mixed, and the issue has not yet been studied in a "gold standard" trial (randomized, placebo-controlled).

In the Interim

If you have AMD, ask your physician whether you should be taking the AREDS vitamin formulation. Current or former smokers should not take this formula, because of evidence linking large doses of beta-carotene with lung cancer in smokers. (As an alternative, they will have to put together their own combination of vitamins. It should include cupric oxide, which is needed to counteract the potential side effects of the high dosage of zinc.)

If it is not appropriate for you to take the AREDS supplement, there are steps you can take: Quit smoking, and keep your weight under control. As for nutrition, you will reap the greatest all-around health benefits by eating a heart-healthy diet that includes healthy oils, fish, and a wide variety of fruits and vegetables, notably green leafy vegetables.

What about supplements of omega-3 fatty acids, lutein, and zeaxanthin? Overall, the FDA recommends that consumers should limit omega-3 intake to 3 grams per day, with no more than 2 grams of that coming from supplements. Lutein and zeaxanthin supplements appear to be safe, although the long-term use of them in supplement form has not been evaluated.

Until the results of AREDS II are in, no one knows for sure what these supplements really mean for preventing macular degeneration or slowing its progression. ■

closed-angle glaucoma may require filtration surgery or long-term use of eyedrops.

Age-Related Macular Degeneration

Age-related macular degeneration (AMD) affects the macula—the central, most sensitive part of the retina. In the United States, AMD is the leading cause of severe and irreversible loss of central vision in people over age 40 years, affecting 1.7 million Americans, or

1.47% of people in this age group. This number is expected to reach almost 3 million people by 2020. Severe vision loss is commonly defined as a decline in visual acuity to 20/200 or less. Visual acuity of 20/200 corresponds to being able to see only the big “E” on an eye chart. People with corrected vision of 20/200 or less in both eyes are considered to be legally blind.

The prevalence of severe vision loss from AMD increases with age, and most people with impaired vision from AMD are age 60 or older. Evidence of AMD can be detected in up to one fourth of people over age 65 and one third of those over age 80. About 2% of people age 65 or older are legally blind because of AMD. Fortunately, most cases of AMD do not result in severe vision loss.

ROLE OF THE RETINA

The retina is the light-sensitive layer of nerve tissue that lines the inner eye. It is made up of millions of tiny nerve receptor cells called cones and rods. Light rays reflected from an object are focused by the cornea and lens onto the retina; the cones and rods then send impulses through the optic nerve to the brain in response to the light.

The most sensitive portion of the retina is a small area at its center, called the **macula**. The macula is about one-fiftieth of an inch in diameter and is responsible for central and fine-detail vision. In the middle of the macula is a small indentation, the fovea, which contains the highest concentration of cones (the most sensitive receptors of light) and provides the sharpest vision. When you look directly at an object, the light rays focus onto the fovea.

Central and detailed vision require an intact macula. If function of the macula is lost, the eye must rely on peripheral vision, which is far less sensitive. As a result, activities such as reading normal-sized print are impossible without the use of low-vision aids.

TYPES OF AGE-RELATED MACULAR DEGENERATION

There are two types of age-related macular degeneration: nonneovascular AMD and neovascular AMD. Sometimes people have both forms at the same time, in one or both eyes. It is also not uncommon for a person with one form to develop the other form later. The onset and progression of either type of AMD do not follow any particular pattern. In its earliest stages, AMD can therefore be difficult to diagnose.

Coping With Drug Costs

Explore your options to pinch pennies

Despite consumer complaints and government hearings, skyrocketing prescription drug prices show no sign of slowing down.

According to an AARP policy report released last spring, the rate of general inflation was 2.3% during the 12-month period of September 2003 to September 2004. But during that same year, drug companies' prices for the 197 brand-name prescription drugs most commonly used by older Americans increased by 7.4%, on average.

Many Americans, especially those older than age 65 years, simply can't keep up. They cope by splitting pills, using eye drops once a day instead of twice as prescribed, or even waiting to refill prescriptions.

If this describes you, take heart: Resources do exist for the financially pressed.

Medicare Drug Benefit

The new federal drug benefit for Medicare enrollees went into effect January 1, 2006, and open enrollment continues until May 16, 2006. Those who qualify for the program will pay no or reduced premiums and deductibles, as well as low co-payments for prescriptions, depending on their incomes and circumstances.

If you have received previous assistance from an individual state or drug company program, you will need to check with those programs, as states and companies are reassessing payment in light of the federal program.

In addition, if the federal program turns you down, you may still be eligible for extra help from your state or from a drug company. This is because income requirements vary among programs.

Other Resources

For more information, here are some additional resources to check out:

AARP. AARP is leading a major campaign against rising prescription drug costs. For information on all aspects of the initiative and frequent updates, go to www.aarp.org/bulletin and click on "prescription drugs" in the upper left-hand navigation bar, or call 888-677-2277.

EyeCare America. EyeCare America, the public service foundation of the American Academy of Ophthalmology, publishes a pharmaceutical directory that lists free or discount ophthalmic drugs available from major drug companies. Drugs on the list include such mainstays of glaucoma treatment as brimonidine (Alphagan P), bimatoprost (Lumigan), timolol (Timoptic), and latanoprost (Xalatan). Each separate drug entry has additional information about income and other eligibility requirements, and how to apply. You will need to consult your physician as part of the application process. For more information, go to www.eyecareamerica.org and click on "assistance with medications," or call 800-222-3937.

Drug companies. Seven drug companies joined together to form Together Rx, offering prescription drug discounts to Medicare enrollees who lack coverage and have incomes below $28,000 ($38,000 for couples). Two caveats: Only one of the 7 companies, Novartis, has ophthalmic drugs. In addition, some of the participating companies may no longer honor the Together Rx program now that the federal program is up and running. (Together Rx is structured so that companies can choose whether or not to continue their involvement.) For more information, call 800-865-7211 or go to www.togetherrx.com.

Three drug companies—Eli Lilly, Merck, and Pfizer—have their own separate programs:

- Eli Lilly: call 877-795-4559 or go to www.lillyanswers.com.
- Merck: call 800-506-3723 or go to www.merckhelps.com.
- Pfizer: call 800-717-6005 or go to www.pfizerforliving.com and click on "Pfizer helpful answers."

NeedyMeds. This resource provides a clearinghouse of information on state and local assistance programs as well as the drug companies' discount prescription programs. Go to www.needymeds.com or call 215-625-9689.

Talk to Your Doctor

It's critical that you follow your medication regimen as prescribed. But eye doctors are well aware that people don't always follow instructions and that drug cost can be a significant barrier to compliance. A recent review confirmed that noncompliance was common in glaucoma care, with up to 80% of glaucoma patients in some studies reporting that they deviate from their prescribed drug regimen.

If this is the case for you, it's time to come clean with your ophthalmologist and discuss your concerns. For one thing, your doctor may have suggestions about which pharmacies in your area offer better prices. (Some physicians have even prepared cost comparison sheets for patients for commonly prescribed ophthalmic drugs.) He or she may also have ideas about treatment alternatives, particularly surgery. Under Medicare and Medicaid coverage, for instance, copayment costs may be more generous for surgery than they are for medication. With glaucoma, in particular, that can make a significant difference, given that a year's worth of medication can run $3,000 or more, while a surgical procedure may be $1,000. ■

Non-neovascular AMD (also known as nonexudative, atrophic, or dry AMD) is the most common; 90% of people with AMD have this type. Non-neovascular AMD is usually characterized by shrinkage of tissues in the retina and formation of drusen, which are small accumulations of debris underneath the retina.

Although this form of AMD cannot be prevented or reversed, the disease progresses slowly and may stabilize for periods of time. In fact, in many people with non-neovascular AMD, vision is not seriously impaired.

In people with non-neovascular AMD, neovascular AMD may develop at any time. The chance of this happening is greater in those who have more or larger drusen and more changes in the pigment epithelial layer (the membrane cellular issue) in the macula.

Neovascular AMD (also called exudative or wet AMD) is the more serious form of the disorder and is the primary cause of AMD-related vision loss. Loss of vision from neovascular AMD occurs either when:

- New blood vessels grow (called neovascularization) from the choroid layer of the eye (the layer between the retina and sclera). These new blood vessels tend to leak fluid under the retina.
- Degeneration of the layer of retinal pigment epithelial cells (cells that contribute to a number of retinal functions) just beneath the retina.

People with neovascular AMD in one eye have up to a 60% chance that the other eye will become similarly affected within 5 years.

Neovascular AMD is further classified by where the new blood vessels are located and by the pattern of fluid leakage. The location of the neovascularization is described in terms of its proximity to the fovea. New vessels farthest away from the fovea are termed extrafoveal; those at the fovea itself are called subfoveal; and those in between are named juxtafoveal.

The pattern of fluid leakage is described as classic (in which the blood vessels involved can easily be seen on exam) or occult (the blood vessels involved are harder to locate). When examined by fluorescein angiography (see "Diagnosing Age-Related Macular Degeneration," pages 39–41), classic new blood vessels tend to be seen leaking more than occult new blood vessels in the early images generated by the test. In addition, the extent of the leakage tends to be defined more clearly with classic new blood vessels compared to occult new blood vessels.

CAUSES OF AGE-RELATED MACULAR DEGENERATION

The causes of both non-neovascular and neovascular AMD are unknown. There are, however, known risk factors for both forms. Increasing age, farsightedness, cigarette smoking, a light-colored iris, and a family history of the disorder all raise the risk for both types. In addition, high blood pressure appears to be linked to a greater risk of neovascular AMD.

A defect in a gene called ABCR may also contribute to AMD. One study found that 16% of people with AMD had a defect in this gene, compared with only 0.5% of people in the general population without AMD. ABCR controls the production of an important protein found in the rods of the retina.

SYMPTOMS OF AGE-RELATED MACULAR DEGENERATION

In most cases, AMD produces no symptoms. When symptoms do occur in people with non-neovascular AMD, they develop gradually. In contrast, symptoms can be severe and occur in a matter of days or weeks in people with neovascular AMD.

Symptoms of AMD include a grayness, haziness, or blank spot in central vision. Words on a page may be blurred, straight lines may appear to have a kink in them, and objects may seem smaller than they are. In addition, color vision may become dimmer because the receptors involved in distinguishing colors (cones) are most dense in the fovea.

People can monitor themselves for AMD-related vision changes using an Amsler grid—a diagram of a box subdivided into many smaller boxes. To use an Amsler grid, hold the grid at reading distance, fix one eye on its center, and cover the other eye. Minor blurring or wavy or distorted lines may indicate early AMD. People with more advanced cases of AMD will have gray areas or blind spots around the center of the grid. Bear in mind that the Amsler grid alone is not a reliable indicator of AMD (see "New Research" column to the right). It is important to monitor your vision during normal activities as well, such as reading and watching television.

PREVENTING AGE-RELATED MACULAR DEGENERATION

Some studies indicate that people can take steps to prevent AMD or slow its progression. These steps include taking dietary supplements and improving overall diet. Reducing exposure to sunlight possibly

NEW RESEARCH

An Alternative to the Amsler Grid

Despite its flaws, the Amsler grid is still in use for early screening of macular degeneration. But more effective screening devices are in development.

One is the preferential hyperacuity perimetry (PHP) device. In a study of 150 people, the PHP device was found to be more sensitive in detecting AMD-related lesions than the Amsler grid. Of 117 people who were determined to have AMD during an examination, 68% had positive results with the PHP device.

In comparison, 26% had positive results with the Amsler grid. One limitation: The PHP device also had a high rate of false-positive results for healthy patients.

The PHP looks like a computer screen. When a person sits in front of it, he or she is instructed to indicate areas that seem distorted on the touch-sensitive screen. As the person indicates any perceived areas of distortion, the PHP software separates these areas into those that are artificial vs. those that are representative of pathology. Responses consistent with neovascular AMD are noted.

RETINA
Volume 25, page 296
April-May 2005

may help as well.

The effect of dietary supplements on the risk and progression of AMD was investigated in the Age-Related Eye Disease Study, which included more than 3,500 people ages 55–80. For an average of 6 years, participants took dietary supplements containing antioxidants, zinc, or antioxidants plus zinc or a placebo. None of the dietary supplements reduced the risk of developing AMD. But in those with intermediate or advanced AMD, the supplement containing antioxidants plus zinc reduced the risk of more advanced AMD by about 25%.

The antioxidant plus zinc supplement used in the study contained 500 mg of vitamin C, 400 IU of vitamin E, 15 mg of beta-carotene, 80 mg of zinc oxide, and 2 mg of cupric oxide. It is sold under the brand name Ocuvite PreserVision and is available without a prescription. If you smoke, or have recently quit, do not use this supplement, because beta-carotene in supplement form has been found to increase the risk of lung cancer in smokers.

Other studies have suggested that eating fruits and vegetables high in carotenoids, especially those high in beta-carotene (carrots, spinach, and cantaloupes, for example), might help prevent AMD. In addition, some studies have found that avoiding excessive exposure to sunlight is protective. In the Beaver Dam Eye Study, people who spent at least 5 hours a day outside during summers when in their teens and 30s had twice the rate of AMD as those who were outside less than 2 hours a day. In addition, those who wore hats and sunglasses tended to have a lower rate of AMD.

Based on these findings, it is probably worthwhile to protect your eyes from UV rays by wearing sunglasses and a wide-brimmed hat when outdoors. Eating plenty of fruits and vegetables rich in carotenoids is probably also protective. Taking vitamin and mineral supplements, however, will not help prevent AMD in healthy people or protect against the progression of AMD in people with early AMD. But people with intermediate or advanced AMD may benefit from these supplements and should ask their doctor about them.

Currently, some clinical trials are testing whether low-powered laser treatment can help prevent AMD. In addition, a large study is investigating whether injections of the drug anecortave acetate can prevent new blood vessel growth before it begins.

Other suspected risk factors for AMD include high cholesterol, obesity, and coronary heart disease. While the degree of their impact is still unclear, it's worth taking steps to improve these factors because of their overall impact on your health.

New Drug for AMD

Fresh promise in pharmaceuticals

Late last year, the FDA approved pegaptanib sodium (Macugen) for the treatment of neovascular macular degeneration.

What makes pegaptanib sodium different from current treatments for neovascular AMD, particularly photodynamic therapy with verteporfin (Visudyne)? Photodynamic therapy is restricted to certain subsets of people with AMD. And while it can help treat pre-existing abnormal blood vessels, it can't prevent new vessels from forming. In contrast, Macugen can be used in a wider range of patients, and it strikes at the molecular level to get at the underlying cause of the disease.

Even so, Macugen isn't the perfect therapy for AMD, and challenges remain.

How It Works

Macugen works by blocking vascular endothelial growth factor (VEGF) in the eye. This protein has a number of positive functions in the body— it helps preserve visual clarity in the healthy eye and it is also needed for normal wound healing and bone growth.

But VEGF also stimulates or induces the process of angiogenesis (when new blood vessels develop from preexisting ones). Angiogenesis is implicated in a number of diseases, most notably cancer.

In the eye, VEGF is a key factor involved in neovascularization and vascular permeability—that is, the proliferation of new vessels that are prone to leakage. Basic science research in the laboratory has shown that when VEGF levels are increased, vessels grow in the retina and choroids. Conversely, blocking VEGF stopped new vessel growth and reduced the likelihood of vessel leakage. This gave AMD researchers the rationale for pursuing drugs that could inhibit VEGF.

Study results. The FDA approved Macugen based on results from 2 randomized, placebo-controlled trials of 1,208 people with neovascular AMD. The participants were given either an injection of placebo or an injection of Macugen (either 0.3-mg, 1-mg, or 3-mg doses) every 6 weeks over a 54-week period. Although the majority of those participating in the study continued to lose vision no matter which treatment they received, moderate and severe vision loss was significantly reduced in those who received Macugen. Those who received 0.3 mg of Macugen did the best overall, with fewer people in this group experiencing severe vision loss.

Potential problems. Because Macugen is given by intravitreal injection, this raises the risk of endophthalmitis (a potentially blinding infection), retinal detachment, and traumatic (injection-caused) cataract. While these risks were minimal during the study, the long-term risk of a series of injections is unclear. In addition, the cost is approximately $995 per injection. With a 6-week injection schedule, that amounts to approximately $8,600 per year per person.

Looking Forward

Macugen isn't the only drug that targets VEGF in the eye. Ranibizumab (Lucentis), which is not yet on the market, also inhibits VEGF. But Lucentis takes a shotgun approach, binding all forms of VEGF (including those thought to be beneficial elsewhere in the body), while Macugen targets VEGF 165 (thought to be the most destructive form of VEGF). Only time will tell which approach will be more effective.

In any case, the issue of repeated injections is still a problematic one. One potential way to reduce the potential for injection-related complications would be to give people with AMD tiny implants that deliver the drugs in a continuous, slow release over several months. Researchers are hot on this trail as well. ■

DIAGNOSING AGE-RELATED MACULAR DEGENERATION

Ophthalmoscopy is used to diagnose non-neovascular AMD. To perform ophthalmoscopy, the doctor dilates your pupils with eyedrops and uses an ophthalmoscope—a special instrument with a light at the end—to magnify and examine the back of your eye. Non-neovascular AMD is diagnosed when the doctor sees drusen or other pigment changes in the macula.

A diagnosis of neovascular AMD is suspected when a person experiences new symptoms and ophthalmoscopy shows leakage of

Herbs and Your Eyes

Even natural remedies have side effects

Are you taking herbal remedies or nutritional supplements for your eye health? If so, it's important to be aware of the potential for side effects.

Late last year, a study that included case reports submitted to the National Registry of Drug-Induced Ocular Side Effects highlighted several adverse ocular effects linked to the use of certain herbal and nutritional supplements.

The side effects ranged from eye dryness to retinal hemorrhages and temporary loss of vision. In most cases, side effects were associated with higher doses of the particular herb or supplement, and they cleared up once the person stopped taking the supplement in question.

Problem Herbs and Supplements

The study linked the following 8 herbs and supplements to clinically significant ocular side effects:

1. Canthaxanthin. This carotenoid is found naturally in certain foods, particularly shellfish and chanterelle mushrooms. It's used as a coloring to add an orange-red hue to foods, in cosmetics and in animal feed. It's also found in "sunless" tanning pills. If taken in large doses , which often happens with the tanning pills, the canthaxanthin is deposited in all layers of the retina. Although the deposits seem to gradually be absorbed by the body, traces of them can take many years to disappear. While most people don't notice any effects linked to the deposits, some people report diminished sharpness of their vision, and changes have been noted on several ophthalmic tests, including electroretinography, which tests how the retina works. These changes are reversible once the body absorbs the canthaxanthin deposits.

2. Chamomile (*Matricaria chamomilla*). Chamomile is often used to treat insomnia, indigestion, and skin problems. Some herbalists also recommend it for styes (infection of one or more of the glands at the edge of the eyelid or under it). However, when applied topically around the eye, as in chamomile tea "washes" or compresses, chamomile can cause severe conjunctivitis (inflammation of the conjunctiva). The author of the study suggested that this might be an allergic reaction to chamomile.

3. Datura (*Datura stramonium and D. wrightii*). This supplement is sometimes used to treat asthma, bronchitis, and coughs. Its ocular side effects include dilated pupils (known as mydriasis) and infection of the cornea (keratitis) which may occur when a person accidentally touches a part of the plant, such as the leaves, and then rubs his or her eyes. Overall, datura isn't commonly used in herbal medicine, given its track record of fatal poisonings. Nonetheless, many datura varieties remain on the market in plant nurseries across the country. In addition, some varieties are indigenous to the Southwestern United States and thus can be found growing in people's yards and public areas.

4. Echinacea (*Echinacea purpurea*). This top-selling herb is used primarily to treat upper respiratory infections. Like chamomile, it's also recommended for styes and can cause eye irritation and conjunctivitis when used topically. And as with chamomile, an allergic reaction may be to blame.

5. Ginkgo (*Ginkgo biloba*). This supplement is extremely popular, used to boost memory and to treat a number of conditions, including

fluid or blood in the area of the macula. The diagnosis is then confirmed by fluorescein angiography, which enables the doctor to closely examine the blood vessels in the eye. This test should be performed and interpreted promptly because neovascular AMD can progress within days.

Fluorescein angiography involves an injection of a dye called fluorescein into a vein in your arm. As the dye circulates and reaches the blood vessels of the eye, photographs of the retina are taken with a special camera. The light from the camera flash passes through a blue filter, and the resulting blue light stimulates the fluorescein to emit a yellow-green light. This allows the doctor to view the fluorescein in the blood vessels of the retina and choroids, and to see if any of the dye has leaked from damaged vessels.

asthma, tinnitus, vertigo, and varicose veins. Some herbalists also recommend it as a treatment for glaucoma and macular degeneration. However, ginkgo's blood-thinning properties have been linked to case reports of bleeding, and some people who have taken the herb have experienced spontaneous hyphema (bleeding in the anterior chamber of the eye) and retinal hemorrhages.

6. Licorice (*Glycyrrhiza glabra*). Licorice is often used to treat a variety of conditions, including respiratory tract infections and constipation. However, it can cause temporary loss of vision, with visual symptoms similar to those of an ocular migraine without headache (double vision and distorted images). While the side effects of licorice appeared to be associated with large doses, smaller doses could potentially trigger the same symptoms in people who are predisposed to develop migraines.

7. Niacin. In tablet form, niacin is used to treat cardiovascular and cerebrovascular disease. It also can be found in certain foods, including red meat. Niacin intake, especially at higher doses, causes a number of ocular side effects, including decreased vision, blurred vision, dry eyes, swollen eyelids, and a condition that resembles cystoid macular edema (swelling of the macula) called pseudo-cystoid macular edema. While the pseudo-cystoid macular edema occurs primarily in people who take more than 3 grams of niacin per day, it has been seen in those taking as little as 1.5 gram per day. Once the person stops taking the niacin, the condition usually clears up within 2 weeks.

8. Vitamin A. This vitamin is so important to health that you'd be hard-pressed to find a daily vitamin supplement without it. The daily recommended intake of vitamin A is 5,000 IU for men and 4,000 IU for women. And more is not better: High doses can cause intracranial hypertension, a condition in which the pressure of the cerebrospinal fluid in the brain rises to an unsafe level. The optic nerve is commonly affected in intracranial hypertension, and blindness is a very real possibility. Fortunately, in the majority of cases reviewed in the study, the intracranial hypertension resolved when the vitamin A was discontinued.

Herbal Interactions

With some of these herbs, there are data on interactions with other medications or cautions about discontinuing them before surgery.

For instance, ginkgo interacts with haliperodol (Haldol), and it can increase the side-effects of antidepressants and certain antibiotics . And because it's a blood thinner, you have a greater risk of bleeding when you take it with other blood thinners, such as aspirin or warfarin (Coumadin). Ginkgo also increases the risk of bleeding during surgery.

As for licorice, do not take it if you are taking a diuretic, digoxin (Lanoxin and others), or insulin.

If you are facing eye surgery (or any other type of surgery), be sure to tell your physician which supplements you are taking. While the recommended time for discontinuing a product before surgery varies, it's safe to stop taking herbs and other supplements 2 weeks before surgery. That should allow enough time for the product to clear your body, thus decreasing the likelihood of any drug interactions or other side effects, including problems with anesthesia.

The bottom line: Any product that has a therapeutic effect can also have a side effect. Herbs are no exception. ■

Fluorescein angiography is associated with serious risks: death in about 1 in 225,000 people and major complications in 1 in 2,000 people. There is also a small chance of nausea or vomiting. But the test is essential to diagnose neovascular AMD and to identify the sites of neovascularization.

A newer test, indocyanine green angiography, which uses a similar procedure but a different dye, may be used if fluorescein angiography does not adequately highlight the abnormal vessels. The green dye can sometimes provide a clear image despite barriers such as bleeding or changes in pigmentation.

People with cataracts may need to have them removed before diagnosis or treatment of AMD, since the cataracts can obstruct the view of the back of the eye. In some cases, removal of the cataracts improves vision.

TREATING AGE-RELATED MACULAR DEGENERATION

Non-neovascular AMD is usually not treated. Instead, people are monitored for the possible development of neovascular AMD. Based on results from the Age-Related Eye Disease Study, people with intermediate non-neovascular AMD in one or both eyes or advanced non-neovascular AMD in one eye might consider taking supplemental antioxidants and zinc to slow the progression of the disease. As mentioned previously, these supplements are available commercially in a product called Ocuvite PreserVision. Check with your doctor before taking any supplements.

Neovascular AMD, in some cases, can be treated with some of the treatments listed below.

Photocoagulation

The standard treatment for neovascular AMD in which new blood vessel growth is not found directly under the fovea is coagulation of the blood vessels with a laser. This procedure, photocoagulation, is noninvasive and is performed on an outpatient basis by an ophthalmologist with special training and experience. It takes about 15–20 minutes. Before the procedure, the pupil is dilated with eyedrops and anesthetized with drops or an injection. The doctor then aims a high-energy laser beam at the new blood vessels to destroy them.

According to the Macular Photocoagulation Study, the procedure decreases the risk of vision loss when well-defined new blood vessels can be identified in extrafoveal, juxtafoveal, or subfoveal sites. For example, in the study participants with extrafoveal AMD, severe vision loss occurred after 18 months in 60% of untreated eyes but in only 25% of treated eyes. The risk of severe vision loss was also lowered after photocoagulation of juxtafoveal and subfoveal vessels. Although benefits of photocoagulation lasted 5 years, they did diminish over time. Recurrence of neovascularization after successful photocoagulation was 10% after 1–2 months, 24% after 6 months, and 54% after 3 years.

Because of this high rate of recurrence of new blood vessel growth after photocoagulation, anyone who has the procedure needs to be carefully monitored, periodically undergoing fluorescein angiography. If new symptoms of vision loss or distortion appear, an immediate examination is needed. A close watch must be maintained on the other eye as well. Some people use an Amsler grid for self-monitoring, but this method is not particularly reliable.

NEW RESEARCH

Macular Degeneration and Cardiovascular Disease

The hypothesis that age-related macular degeneration and heart disease share some common ground received additional support from a study of cardiovascular biomarkers and AMD progression.

In a prospective study of 251 people with AMD, researchers measured the blood levels of several indicators of inflammation. The biomarkers are all known to play a role in the development of cardiovascular disease, and earlier studies have raised the possibility that they might play a role in AMD as well.

Of the 251 people, 96 progressed to advanced stages of AMD. And 2 of the biomarkers, C-reactive protein (CRP) and interleukin-6 (IL-6), were found to significantly increase this risk of progression. Those who had the highest levels of CRP and IL-6 experienced a 2-fold greater risk of progression than those who had the lowest levels. This increased risk held even after the researchers ruled out other factors known to increase the risk of AMD progression, such as smoking and obesity.

Reducing CRP and IL-6 levels might have a favorable impact on the progression rate of AMD, the researchers note. One potential treatment would be statin medications, which are commonly used for heart disease. However, more research on the use of statins in AMD is needed, as previous studies have come up with conflicting results.

ARCHIVES OF OPHTHALMOLOGY
Volume 123, page 774
June 2005

The major potential complication of photocoagulation is damage to the macula, which can result in a permanent blind spot in the center of the visual field. This complication is most common in people with neovascularization close to or at the center of the macula.

Photodynamic Therapy

A newer option for treating neovascular AMD is photodynamic therapy, which was approved by the FDA in 2000. The procedure is particularly helpful for people who have neovascularization directly under the fovea but cannot undergo photocoagulation because of their high risk of vision loss.

Photodynamic therapy is a 2-step procedure performed in a doctor's office. It involves injecting a light-sensitive drug called verteporfin (Visudyne) into the arm. The drug has a preference for binding to cells in the new blood vessels. The doctor then beams a low-powered laser into the eye to activate the drug, which destroys abnormal tissue but leaves normal tissue intact. As a result, growth of abnormal vessels stops, and vision loss is stabilized with minimal damage to the retina.

In randomized trials led by researchers at Johns Hopkins, 402 patients with neovascularization received photodynamic therapy and 207 patients received placebo therapy. After 2 years, 53% of the people in the photodynamic group had no further vision loss, compared with 38% of those in the placebo group. In the third year, further vision loss in the photodynamic group was minimal, particularly in people with predominantly classic neovascularization. Adverse side effects of photodynamic therapy included pain, swelling, hemorrhage, and inflammation at the injection site. Photosensitivity reactions were seen in about 1% of the participants.

Pegaptanib

A drug called pegaptanib (Macugen) blocks the action of a protein called vascular endothelial growth factor (VEGF), which promotes the growth of new blood vessels in the eye. The FDA approved pegaptanib in late 2004, making it the first treatment for neovascular AMD that can be used in a wide range of people with the disease. (See "New Drug for AMD" on page 39 for more information on pegaptanib.)

When any of these therapies are ineffective or cannot be performed, low-vision aids can often help with daily activities, despite vision loss in both eyes. Researchers are also working on a number

NEW RESEARCH

NSAIDs May Cut Macular Degeneration Risk

In an unexpected finding, a study of people with rheumatoid arthritis found that they had a much lower incidence of macular degeneration. The reason? Long-term treatment with nonsteroidal inflammatory drugs (NSAIDs), the researchers suggest.

In a study conducted in Canada, the incidence of AMD was assessed in 993 people over the age of 65 years. All had been followed closely since they were initially diagnosed with rheumatoid arthritis in their 50s.

The researchers found only 3 cases of AMD. In comparison, previous population studies have suggested that they could have expected to find approximately 30 cases of AMD.

Long-term use of NSAIDs may lower AMD incidence, the researchers say, and the finding supports the developing hypothesis that AMD is an inflammatory disease. They also note that genetic or environmental factors could also be responsible for the much lower rate seen in these arthritis patients.

NEUROBIOLOGY OF AGING
Volume 26, page 1199
August-September 2005

of new drugs and surgical procedures that may one day prove beneficial for people with neovascular AMD.

Experimental Treatments

Several new treatments that may help prevent vision loss—or even improve vision—in people with AMD are under investigation. Another VEGF-blocking drug, ranibizumab (Lucentis), is being studied, as are drugs known as angiostatic corticosteroids (such as anecortave acetate, triamcinolone, and flucinolone). These treatments may help prevent new blood vessel growth as well as leakage from blood vessels in the eye. Other treatments that researchers are working on include radiation therapy, thermotherapy, and surgery.

New surgical techniques are also under development. In one procedure called subfoveal surgery, which is being studied at Johns Hopkins and other medical centers, abnormal new blood vessels are surgically removed from behind the retina. While early results appeared promising, more recent reports indicate that the procedure does not stabilize or improve vision.

Several years ago, researchers at Johns Hopkins began investigating macular translocation, a surgical technique to move the retina. In people with subfoveal neovascularization, the retina is detached, moved, and reattached so that the subfoveal vessels become extrafoveal, where they then can be treated with photocoagulation without harming central vision. Early results showed improvement in up to one third of study participants. Interest in macular translocation has dwindled since the advent of photodynamic therapy, however.

Low-Vision Aids

In people with AMD, low-vision aids can help optimize remaining vision and improve the ability to perform daily activities. Some examples of low-vision aids are telescopes, closed-circuit televisions (a small television camera mounted on a movable tray; documents or other objects are moved under the camera and viewed on a small monitor), magnifying glasses, clocks and phones with large numbers, and large-print reading materials. Telescopes and closed-circuit televisions require an evaluation and prescription from an eye care professional, as well as training in how to use them. Many low-vision aids are available through low-vision clinics and low-vision rehabilitation services.

NEW RESEARCH

Dry Eye and Diabetes

People with diabetes, especially those with poor glycemic control, are more likely than non-diabetic patients to have dry eye.

Researchers followed the medical records of 159,624 people who belonged to an Israeli HMO for 1 year. All of the participants were older than age 50, and 22,382 had diabetes.

The researchers tracked the use of artificial tears among the patients with diabetes and those who did not have the disorder. At the end of the year, 20.6% of the patients with diabetes and 13.8% of those without diabetes had used artificial tears. Moreover, the researchers found a clear trend of greater use of artificial tears as glycemic control (measured by levels of HbA1c) declined.

The researchers note that dry eye in people with diabetes may be due in part to damage to the microvasculature of the lacrimal gland (which secretes tears) in the eye. Sensory neuropathy (a nerve disorder) in the cornea also may play a role, as may side effects of medications used to control diabetes.

AMERICAN JOURNAL OF OPHTHALMOLOGY
Volume 139, page 498
March 2005

Hypertension and the Eye

High blood pressure can threaten your vision

While many people are aware that diabetes can damage the retina, they may not know that hypertension can threaten their vision as well.

The most common ocular sign of chronic hypertension is narrowing of the tiny retinal vessels. As hypertension progresses, retinal vein hemorrhages and blockages may occur.

Regular eye exams can pick up the early signs of retinal damage in someone who already has hypertension. But they may also help flag people who are at increased risk of developing severe hypertension down the line.

For instance, in the Atherosclerosis Risk in Communities study, a population-based study conducted in 4 U.S. communities, researchers took photographs of participant's retinas and identified areas of arteriolar narrowing. After 3 years of follow-up, they found that the risk of new-onset hypertension was 60% higher in people whose retinal photographs showed narrowing of the retinal vessels than in those who did not have any evidence of retinal changes. In addition, the arteriolar narrowing turned out to be a separate risk factor for hypertension, independent of established risk factors such as obesity.

Two additional studies, one from Australia and a second from the United States, confirmed the finding that people with small changes in the walls of their retinal vessels had a higher chance of developing hypertension.

In a long-running eye study in Australia, people with narrowed retinal arterioles were more than twice as likely to develop severe hypertension in 5 years than were those without such changes. Again, changes in retinal vessels were an independent risk factor for hypertension, separate from other risk factors such as age, obesity, smoking, and blood glucose levels. Changes in retinal vessels were also independent of participant's blood pressure readings when the study began.

In a long-running eye study in Wisconsin called the Beaver Dam Study, arteriolar narrowing was linked to a 3-fold higher risk of developing hypertension over a 10-year period.

Taken together, these studies provide strong evidence that microvascular changes in the eye may be used to flag people who are at greater risk of developing hypertension. They also remind us that regular eye exams are essential, both for monitoring the health of our eyes and for keeping tabs on systemic diseases.

Hypertension and Glaucoma

It is probably not surprising to learn that increased blood pressure in the body is linked to increased intraocular pressure (IOP).

Evidence that this is indeed the case came from the Beaver Dam eye study. Over a 5-year period in which participants' systemic blood pressure and IOP readings were monitored, the researchers found that every increase of 10 mm Hg in systolic blood pressure (the top number in your blood pressure reading) was linked to an average increase of 0.21 mm Hg in IOP (normal eye pressures range from about 10 to 21 mm Hg.) In addition, every increase of 10 mm Hg in diastolic blood pressure (the bottom number in your blood pressure reading) led to an average increase of 0.43 mm Hg in IOP.

Conversely, decreases in systolic or diastolic blood pressure were associated with drops in IOP. Thus, if you have glaucoma, it's worth making efforts to get your blood pressure under control. Every bit counts.

Hypertension and Diabetes

Not only can those narrowed retinal vessels predict an increased risk of developing hypertension, they also can predict whether someone is at risk of developing type 2 diabetes.

In another Beaver Dam study, people who had narrowed arterioles were more likely to develop diabetes over a 10-year period. And hypertension just added to the risk: Those who had both hypertension and narrowed arterioles had a 3-fold higher risk of developing diabetes than those whose blood pressure stayed normal and who had no retinal vascular changes.

If you've already been diagnosed with diabetes, controlling your blood pressure is critical for preventing diabetic retinopathy or slowing its progression.

In a series of reports from a long-running eye study conducted in the United Kingdom, intensive treatment of diabetes, which included tight control of blood pressure in addition to blood glucose levels, prevented and reduced the progression of microvascular complications in the eye.

The researchers note that high blood pressure increases blood flow in the eye, thus increasing "shear stress" in the retinal vasculature. This damages the vessels' walls and both precipitates and worsens diabetic retinopathy.

Again, whether you already have diabetes or are worried about developing it, controlling your blood pressure is key to safeguarding your overall health and the health of your eyes. ■

Diabetic Retinopathy

About 18 million Americans have diabetes, a condition characterized by abnormally high levels of glucose (sugar) in the blood. Although no cure exists for diabetes, blood glucose levels can be controlled by carefully following a program of diet, exercise, and (if necessary) medication.

High blood glucose levels can damage small blood vessels in the retina, a condition called diabetic retinopathy. The condition affects more than 4.1 million Americans age 40 and over and is more common in people with poorly controlled diabetes. Nearly 900,000 Americans have diabetic retinopathy severe enough to cause vision loss.

CAUSES OF DIABETIC RETINOPATHY

There are two forms of diabetes: type 1 and type 2. In type 1 diabetes, mild abnormalities in the retina begin to appear an average of 7 years after the diabetes begins, but damage that threatens vision usually does not develop until much later. In people with type 2 diabetes—the more common type—retinopathy may be present at the time of diagnosis or relatively soon afterward. This is because the onset of type 2 diabetes is gradual, and changes in the retina may have already taken place before the diabetes is even diagnosed. Almost all people with type 1 diabetes will eventually develop retinopathy, compared with 70% of those with type 2 diabetes. However, people with type 2 diabetes are less likely to develop more advanced retinopathy than those with type 1. Currently, an estimated 32% of people age 18 and older who were diagnosed with type 1 diabetes before they turned 30 have vision-threatening retinopathy.

Microaneurysms. In the early, or nonproliferative, stages of diabetic retinopathy, blood vessels in the retina develop weak spots that bulge outward (microaneurysms) and may leak fluid and blood into the surrounding retinal tissue. These initial abnormalities usually cause no visual symptoms, and in many people the disease progresses no further.

Macular edema. Swelling around the macula (macular edema) caused by the leakage and accumulation of fluid can occur in people with diabetes. The swelling alters the position of the retina and causes blurred vision. Loss of vision is more pronounced when the center of the macula is affected.

Proliferative retinopathy. This is the most dangerous form of

NEW RESEARCH

New Treatment for Dry Eye

Autologous serum eye drops, which are derived from a person's own blood, are gaining ground as a potential treatment for severe dry eye disease that doesn't respond to conventional treatment.

Japanese researchers divided a group of 20 people with severe dry eye disease into 2 subsets. One used only preservative-free artificial tears and the second used only autologous serum eye drops for 2 weeks of treatment.

At the end of the treatment period, those who had used the autologous eye drops showed significant improvement on several clinical measures of the health of the eye's surface and reported greater improvement on subjective measures of comfort.

Autologous serum eye drops, contain essential tear components, such as vitamin A and several growth factors. They have been found to be beneficial in treating several other eye surface diseases.

As for their use in treating dry eye, the researchers say that the next step is to evaluate a larger group of patients over a longer treatment period.

AMERICAN JOURNAL OF OPHTHALMOLOGY
Volume 139, page 242
February 2005

diabetic retinopathy, characterized by neovascularization—the growth of small, new blood vessels onto the back surface of the vitreous humor. Acute loss of vision can occur when the new blood vessels rupture and bleed into the vitreous humor or when scar tissue pulls the retina away from the back of the eye (retinal detachment).

Researchers don't yet understand exactly how high blood glucose levels cause diabetic retinopathy, but a possibility involves a protein known as vascular endothelial growth factor (VEGF) which promotes the growth of new blood vessels in the eye and is secreted into the eye in response to damage caused by diabetes. Studies also suggest that high cholesterol and triglyceride levels as well as high blood pressure can increase the risk of diabetic retinopathy. These conditions are more common in people with diabetes than in the general population.

SYMPTOMS OF DIABETIC RETINOPATHY

The early stages of diabetic retinopathy generally cause no symptoms, so periodic eye exams are necessary to detect the condition. Even proliferative retinopathy does not initially produce symptoms.

Symptoms develop only when there is bleeding in the eye. A person sees spots or showers of small spots called floaters, which can be severe enough to block vision entirely. Sudden bleeding into the vitreous humor can cause rapid vision loss.

Blood vessel changes can cause macular edema or closure of the small vessels supplying the macula (macular nonperfusion), resulting in blurring of vision. Scar tissue on the macula due to proliferative retinopathy can also cause blurry vision.

Retinal detachment symptoms include wavy or watery vision, a dark shadow in part of the peripheral field of vision, and/or sudden blindness in one eye.

PREVENTING DIABETIC RETINOPATHY

If you have diabetes, you can take several steps to prevent diabetic retinopathy from developing or to slow its progression. Precautions include getting regular eye exams and keeping your blood glucose and blood pressure under tight control. Blood glucose levels are considered well controlled when hemoglobin A1c levels are less than 7%.

Two large studies have proven the benefits of controlling blood glucose levels when it comes to eye health. In the Diabetes Control

NEW RESEARCH

Retinopathy and Congestive Heart Failure

Retinopathy (a noninflammatory disorder of the retina) may signify systemic microcirculatory problems that could lead to congestive heart failure (CHF), especially in people who don't have other risk factors for CHF.

In a subset of the Atherosclerosis Risk in Communities Study, retinal photographs were taken in 11,612 people aged 49–73 years. The photographs were evaluated for presence of retinopathy.

During a 7-year follow-up period, 492 people were diagnosed with CHF. Among those who had no other risk factors for CHF (heart disease, diabetes, or hypertension), the presence of retinopathy was associated with a 3-fold higher risk of developing CHF. Those who had retinopathy and other pre-existing CHF risk factors were twice as likely to develop CHF.

Retinopathy is an independent predictor of CHF, the researchers conclude, and they note that if a person is found have retinopathy during an ophthalmic examination, it may be appropriate to refer the person for a cardiovascular workup.

JOURNAL OF THE AMERICAN MEDICAL ASSOCIATION
Volume 293, page 63
January 5, 2005

and Complications Trial, people with type 1 diabetes who gave themselves multiple insulin injections each day reduced the risk of developing diabetic retinopathy by 76% and the risk of their condition getting worse by 54%, compared with people who followed a less rigorous treatment regimen. In the United Kingdom Prospective Diabetes Study, people with type 2 diabetes who controlled their blood glucose levels with medication were 30% less likely to have retinopathy that required laser treatment than people who relied on diet and exercise alone. As for lowering blood pressure, a recent study found that every 10 mm Hg reduction in systolic blood pressure (the top number) decreased the incidence of retinopathy and other diabetic complications by 12%.

Reducing blood pressure may even help people with diabetes who don't have high blood pressure. In a study of people with type 2 diabetes whose blood pressure was below 140/90 mm Hg, lowering blood pressure to about 128/75 mm Hg with medication resulted in less progression of diabetic retinopathy over a 5-year period than that seen in people whose blood pressure averaged 137/81 mm Hg. People with diabetes should keep their blood pressure below 130/80 mm Hg.

Research also suggests that lowering blood cholesterol levels and quitting smoking may be helpful in preventing both the development and progression of diabetic retinopathy.

DIAGNOSING DIABETIC RETINOPATHY

Because diabetic retinopathy often produces no symptoms—even in its advanced stages—and because early treatment of advanced retinopathy can usually stop vision loss, people with diabetes need to visit their ophthalmologist regularly. If you have type 1 diabetes, you should begin seeing an ophthalmologist for annual eye exams no later than 5 years after diabetes is diagnosed. Because significant retinopathy may be present at the time of diagnosis in people with type 2 diabetes, an eye examination by an ophthalmologist is advised immediately and annually thereafter. More frequent exams are needed for people with more advanced retinopathy.

At the exam, the ophthalmologist dilates the pupils with eyedrops and directly views the retina with an ophthalmoscope. The ophthalmologist will look for signs of edema (accumulation of fluid), fluid leakage, new blood vessel growth, bleeding, and other abnormalities. Because the eyedrops cause the eyes to be extremely sensitive to light, you should bring a pair of sunglasses with you and

NEW RESEARCH

Telemedicine and Diabetic Retinopathy

Although people with diabetes are at higher risk for eye problems than the general public, 40% do not have eye exams regularly.

Telemedicine can extend screening into rural areas or otherwise underserved populations. Telemedicine allows taking images of the eye long distance and transmitting them electronically to a designated medical center where trained "readers" assess each image.

Researchers in Boston worked with a Veteran's Administration facility in Maine to study 2,437 eyes of 1,219 patients with diabetes. Most (98.9%) of the patients were male, and 91.6% had type 2 diabetes.

The researchers found that 23.4% of the eyes had some form of diabetic retinopathy (63% had no sign of the disease; 13% of the eyes could not be graded). Also, 2.1% of the eyes had early or clinically significant macular edema (78.3% of the eyes had no evidence of disease and could not be graded.)

The telemedicine program picked up other indications of trouble—58.7% of the patients had at least 1 non-diabetic eye problem severe enough to warrant referral, including macular degeneration, cataract, suspected renal disease or hypertension, and retinal vein occlusion.

The researchers concluded telemedicine can identify the severity of diabetic retinopathy and nondiabetic ocular conditions.

AMERICAN JOURNAL OF OPHTHALMOLOGY
Volume 139, page 597
April 2005

Artificial Vision

New frontiers in sight

For blind people, recovering even the slightest bit of vision would be a revolutionary step. Just being able to see the outline of a doorway would propel them into a different world than that of complete blindness.

We're getting closer to this goal. A number of research teams around the world are working on various versions of the artificial retina, formally known as the intraocular retinal prosthesis.

While the devices are still undergoing rigorous testing and development, two types have been implanted in a handful of people—the Argus and the Artificial Silicon Retina microchip. The results to date have raised hopes as well as cautions.

Some promising news: In recent research conducted in Southern California with the Argus, people who have had the device implanted report that they can see some light and detect objects and motion. This is vision in its most rudimentary form. The 6 people tested were able to distinguish large, simple shapes (such as the capital letter L) 60–80% of the time. They did better with objects and were able to indicate whether a cup, a plate, or a knife had been placed before them.

How They Work

The Argus, which is considered the furthest along in development, has several components. A thin chip with 16 electrodes on it is implanted in the eye, and a second chip is implanted behind the ear. The final component is a pair of sunglasses equipped with a miniature video camera and a microprocessor.

When the person wears the glasses, the video camera captures images and converts them to electrical impulses that are transmitted to the chip behind the ear, which then relays them to the retinal chip. The retinal chip functions in lieu of damaged rods and cones and sends impulses directly to the retinal ganglion cells, which pass them along to the visual cortex of the brain. For each electrode that is stimulated on the chip, the person sees a dot of light. To say that one of the people in the Argus study "sees" a plate or cup, then, means something different than what we think of when we think of vision: They see one or more points of light, perhaps a string of lights, not a formed image. Still, for someone who is blind, this is a thrilling advance.

Other artificial retinas in development around the world are similar in theory to the Argus. But the team developing the Artificial Silicon Retina microchip (ASR) has taken a completely different tack. The ASR—which is implanted in the sub-retinal space, between the pigment epithelial layer of the retina and the outer layer—is powered solely by natural, incident light. As a result, it needs no external source of power.

The surface of the ASR is coated with 5,000 microscopic solar cells. The ASR's developers say that these solar cells convert the light that passes through the eye into electrical currents that stimulate visual signals in remaining functional retinal cells. These signals are then sent by the optic nerve to the brain.

Critics of the ASR question whether light entering the eye is strong enough to power the miniature solar cells and produce any vision at all. However, results with the first 6 people who received the implant showed that all reported improvements in their vision. To date, the ASR has been implanted in more than 20 people.

Both the Argus and the ASR have been implanted in patients with retinitis pigmentosa (RP, a rare, inherited disease that leads to tunnel vision and then blindness) and researchers hope to eventually test them in people with age-related macular degeneration. While RP and AMD damage the structures of the eye that normally convert light to electrical impulses, they spare the neural paths to the brain that transport the electrical signals. People with diseases that damage the optic nerve wouldn't be eligible for the artificial retina.

What's Next?

This research has raised many questions, including the following:

- How much current can the retina tolerate?
- What's the best site for the chip to be implanted in terms of yielding the best perception and requiring the lowest, safest electrical charge needed to stimulate neurons?
- Will the retinal neurons tolerate long-term electrical stimulation without being altered in any way?

Another question researchers have been grappling with is how many light-producing electrodes can fit on a chip without damaging the retina? That is, how do you provide enough power, but not so much that it generates tissue-destroying heat?

The current Argus chip has 16 electrodes. The next step is a 60-electrode model, which began testing last year. The eventual goal is a 1,000-electrode model. Theoretically, a person with this model would be able recognize faces and, perhaps, read again (albeit text that would need to be in very large font sizes).

If all goes well, it's possible that the Argus could be commercially available by 2010. But it won't be inexpensive. Its developers estimate that it could run $30,000–50,000 per person. In addition, those who receive it are likely to need extensive "brain training," as the initial studies have shown that it takes people time to learn how to work with the device and interpret the signals being sent to the brain. ■

may want to ask someone to drive you home afterward. Fluorescein angiography is also used to examine the retina for blood vessel changes.

TREATING DIABETIC RETINOPATHY

Tight blood glucose control lessens the risk that retinopathy will get worse. Treating other conditions, such as high blood pressure and abnormal cholesterol levels, may also slow progression. In most cases, no treatment is required for nonproliferative retinopathy, though the retina is carefully monitored for the development of macular edema or proliferative retinopathy. These two conditions can be treated with laser photocoagulation or vitrectomy.

Laser photocoagulation. Photocoagulation uses lasers to promote closure of new blood vessels, halting or slowing down vision loss in most people if performed before too much damage has already occurred. In people with macular edema, focal laser photocoagulation is performed to target individual blood vessels. There are 2 types:

- Panretinal photocoagulation, which creates a grid-like pattern across a larger area of the retina, is used to treat proliferative retinopathy and causes new blood vessels to regress, cutting the risk of blindness in half in people with proliferative retinopathy.
- Focal laser photocoagulation improves vision in only about 10% of people with macular edema, but even when vision does not improve, the risk of further deterioration is halved.

Although complications are rare, both types of laser photocoagulation carry a risk of vision loss.

Vitrectomy. If the extent or location of the damage makes photocoagulation ineffective, or if the vitreous humor is too clouded with blood, vision can often be improved or stabilized with vitrectomy—a surgical procedure that removes the vitreous humor and replaces it with saline solution. Photocoagulation can also be performed during vitrectomy with a special laser that is inserted into the eye. About 70% of those who undergo vitrectomy notice improvement or stabilization of their vision, and some recover enough vision to resume reading and driving.

Experimental treatments. Several new treatments are being tested for diabetic retinopathy. VEGF is a protein that promotes the growth of new blood vessels in the eye, and leakage from these and other vessels can lead to vision loss in people with diabetic retinopathy. Researchers have therefore focused on developing drugs that block the activity of VEGF. Three VEGF inhibitors—ranibizumab (Lucentis), pegaptanib (Macugen), and a drug known as LY333531—are currently being studied in people with diabetic retinopathy.

Another experimental treatment relies on corticosteroids, which are usually prescribed to relieve pain and inflammation caused by various disorders. However, anecortave, triamcinolone, and flucinolone are corticosteroids that can also prevent new blood vessel growth (called angiostatic corticosteroids) and leakage from blood vessels in the eye. Researchers theorize that these drugs block the growth and movement of cells required for the formation of new blood vessel. They also think these corticosteroids may prevent leakage by preserving the tight spaces between the cells that line blood vessel walls. Like VEGF inhibitors, angiostatic corticosteroids are investigational therapies and are not approved by the FDA. ■

GLOSSARY

A-scan ultrasonography—A test that uses sound waves to measure the length of the eyeball.

accommodating IOL—An implant containing a hinge that allows for both near and far vision, thereby mimicking the movement of the natural lens of a young person.

accommodation—The process by which the natural lens changes shape, allowing it to focus on near or far objects.

adrenergic agonist eyedrops—A treatment for glaucoma. The eyedrops reduce intraocular pressure by decreasing the production of aqueous humor and increasing its drainage through the uveoscleral pathway.

age-related macular degeneration (AMD)—A loss of central vision caused by changes in the macula.

Amsler grid—A diagram of a box subdivided into smaller boxes that is used for self-monitoring by people with AMD.

angiostatic corticosteroids—Drugs being studied for treating AMD and diabetic retinopathy.

antimetabolites—Drugs sometimes used in filtration surgery for glaucoma.

aqueous humor—A watery fluid that is located in front of the lens and provides nutrients to the lens and cornea.

astigmatism—Blurred or distorted vision that is common in nearsighted people.

B-scan ultrasonography—A test that uses sound waves to view structures in the back of the eye.

beta-blocker eyedrops—A treatment for glaucoma. The eyedrops reduce intraocular pressure (IOP) by decreasing the production of aqueous humor.

bifocals—A pair of glasses with lenses that correct both distant and near vision.

body mass index (BMI)—A measure of weight in relation to height. To calculate your BMI, multiply your weight in pounds by 704 and divide that by the square of your height in inches. Overweight is defined as a BMI of 25–29.9; obesity is defined as a BMI of 30 or greater.

carbonic anhydrase inhibitors—Medications used to treat glaucoma. These drugs decrease the production of aqueous humor and are available in both oral and eyedrop formulations.

cataract—A cloudiness (opacification) of the lens that can lead to visual impairment.

central vision—The middle part of the visual field.

choroid—A layer of the eye inside the sclera. It contains a dark pigment that minimizes scattering of light inside the eye.

ciliary body—A part of the eye that surrounds the lens and produces aqueous humor.

classic AMD—One of two types of neovascular AMD. Classification is based on fluid leakage patterns.

closed-angle glaucoma—A type of glaucoma caused by a blockage near the iris that prevents aqueous humor from reaching the trabecular meshwork. It results in a rapid buildup of extremely high intraocular pressure that can lead to severe, permanent vision damage within a couple of days.

cones—Nerve cells in the retina that are activated only in bright light and by the colors red, blue, and green.

conjunctiva—A thin, lubricating mucous membrane that covers the sclera and lines the inside of the eyelid.

cornea—The transparent, dome-shaped disk covering the iris and pupil.

coronary heart disease—Abnormality of the arteries that supply blood and oxygen to the heart and can lead to chest pain or a heart attack.

cortical cataract—A cataract that affects the lens cortex.

cyclodestructive surgery—A treatment for glaucoma that destroys the ciliary body with a laser.

cystoid macular edema—A specific pattern of swelling of the central retina.

diabetes—A disease characterized by abnormally high glucose (sugar) levels in the blood.

diabetic retinopathy—Damage to small blood vessels in the retina resulting from the chronic high blood glucose levels in people with poorly controlled diabetes. Proliferative retinopathy is the most dangerous form.

drusen—Small accumulations of debris underneath the retina.

dry AMD—See non-neovascular AMD.

endophthalmitis—An infection of the vitreous humor that develops in a small number of people after eye surgery.

extracapsular surgery—Cataract surgery that removes the front of the lens capsule along with the cortex and nucleus of the lens, while leaving the back of the lens capsule intact.

extrafoveal blood vessels—See neovascular AMD.

exudative AMD—See neovascular AMD.

farsightedness—See hyperopia.

filtration surgery—A treatment for glaucoma that uses conventional surgical instruments to open a passage through the clogged trabecular meshwork, allowing excess aqueous humor to drain into surrounding tissues.

floaters—Black spots or shapes that drift through the field of vision.

fluorescein angiography—A diagnostic procedure for age-related macular degeneration and other retinal diseases. A special dye, called fluorescein, is injected into a vein in the arm. Photographs of the retina are taken as the dye circulates through the blood vessels of the eye.

fovea—The small indentation at the center of the macula. It contains the highest concentration of cones and provides the sharpest vision.

ganglion cells—A type of cell in the retina. Damage to these cells is thought to play a role in the development of glaucoma.

glare—Light within the field of vision that is brighter than other objects to which the eyes have adapted.

glaucoma—An eye disease that results in damage to the optic nerve. Contrary to popular belief, it is not always caused by elevated intraocular pressure.

gonioscopy—A technique used to distinguish between open- and closed-angle glaucoma. It involves an examination of the front part of the eye to check the angle where the iris meets the cornea.

hemorrhage—Leakage of blood from blood vessels.

hyperopia—Farsightedness. Distant objects can be seen clearly, but close ones do not come into proper focus.

indocyanine green angiography—A test similar to fluorescein angiography, using a different dye.

intracapsular surgery—Cataract surgery that removes the entire lens (the front and back of the lens capsule, the cortex, and nucleus). Rarely performed today.

intraocular lens implant (IOL)—A plastic lens that replaces the lens removed during cataract surgery.

intraocular pressure (IOP)—The pressure exerted by the fluids inside the eyeball.

IOL—See intraocular lens implant.

iridectomy—A treatment for closed-angle glaucoma that involves removing part of the iris.

iridotomy—A treatment for closed-angle glaucoma that creates a hole in the iris with a laser.

iris—The colored circle in the middle of the eye that controls the amount of light that enters the eye.

juxtafoveal blood vessels—See neovascular AMD.

LASEK—This stands for laser-assisted subepithelial keratomileusis, a refractive surgery procedure that reshapes the cornea.

laser trabecular surgery—A treatment for glaucoma that involves making 80–100 tiny laser burns in the area of the trabecular meshwork. The procedure increases the drainage of aqueous humor.

LASIK—This stands for laser-assisted in situ keratomileusis, a refractive surgery procedure that reshapes the cornea.

legal blindness—Vision that is 20/200 or worse in both eyes (20/200 vision is the ability to see at 20 feet what a normal eye can see at 200 feet.)

lens—A transparent, dome-shaped disk that is responsible (along with the cornea) for the eye's ability to focus light.

lens capsule—The outermost structure of the lens.

lens cortex—The second innermost structure of the lens, it surrounds the nucleus, and its outer edge is lined with a layer of cells called the epithelium.

lens epithelium—Cells that line the outer surface of the lens cortex.

lens nucleus—The center structure of the lens. Surrounded by the cortex.

macula—A small area at the center of the retina that is responsible for central and fine-detail vision.

low vision aids—Items that can help people with poor vision. Examples include closed-circuit televisions, magnifying glasses, telephones with large numbers, and large-print reading materials.

macular edema—A swelling of the macula caused by leakage and accumulation of fluid. More common in people with diabetes than in the general population.

macular nonperfusion—Closure of small blood vessels that supply the macula.

microaneurysms—Weak spots that bulge outward from blood vessels, including those of the retina.

miotic eyedrops—Used to treat glaucoma, these eyedrops increase the outflow of aqueous humor through the trabecular meshwork by constricting the pupil.

monofocal IOL—A single-focus lens used after cataract surgery to provide clear distance vision.

monovision—A process in which one eye is corrected for distance and the other for near vision. Achieved with an IOL in cataract surgery, in refractive surgery, or even with contact lenses.

multifocal IOL—A type of lens used after cataract surgery. It contains several rings with a common center that focus and adjust for either near or far vision. This allows the eye to be in focus for near and far vision simultaneously.

myocilin—A protein in trabecular meshwork cells. Mutations in the myocilin gene have been identified as a cause of glaucoma.

GLOSSARY—continued

myopia—Also called nearsightedness, a vision deficit in which close objects can be seen clearly, but distant ones do not come into proper focus.

neovascular age-related macular degeneration—A form of AMD in which new blood vessels grow in the choroid layer of the eye. The blood vessels are classified according to their location—subfoveal blood vessels occur at the fovea, extrafoveal blood vessels are farthest away from the fovea, and juxtafoveal blood vessels are in between.

neovascularization—The growth of new blood vessels.

nonexudative AMD—See non-neovascular AMD.

non-neovascular age-related macular degeneration—A form of AMD characterized by the breakdown or thinning of tissues in the macula and the formation of drusen and shrinkage of tissues in the retina. This form of AMD often does not impair vision.

normal tension glaucoma—A type of glaucoma that results from damage to the optic nerve although intraocular pressure is normal.

nuclear cataract—A cataract affecting the nucleus of the lens.

occult AMD—One of two types of neovascular AMD, classified by fluid leakage patterns. Occult AMD is common but difficult to treat.

opacification—The process of becoming opaque or less penetrable to light. Common in the cornea and lens of the eye in people with glaucoma.

open-angle glaucoma—The most common form of glaucoma. It usually produces no obvious symptoms until late stages.

ophthalmologist—A physician who specializes in the diagnosis and treatment of eye diseases.

ophthalmoscopy—Examination of the interior structures of the eye, especially the retina, using a specialized instrument called an ophthalmoscope.

optic nerve—A nerve at the back of the eye that carries visual information from the retina to the brain.

optineurin—A protein found in the trabecular meshwork and retina. Its role is not fully understood, but defects in the gene that directs its production have been associated with glaucoma.

pegaptanib—A recently approved drug used to treat neovascular AMD. Sold under the name Macugen.

perimetry—A test used to determine a person's visual fields. While the person looks straight ahead at a bowl-shaped white area, a computer generates a light in fixed locations around the bowl. The patient indicates each time he or she sees the light.

peripheral vision—The ability to see objects at the edges of the visual field.

phacoemulsification—A type of extracapsular surgery that is performed with an ultrasonic device that nearly liquefies the nucleus and cortex so that they can be removed by suction through a tube.

photocoagulation—The standard treatment for neovascular AMD when the new blood vessels are outside the center of the retina. The procedure involves closing the new blood vessels with a laser. It is also used to treat diabetic retinopathy. Focal laser photocoagulation targets individual blood vessels; panretinal photocoagulation creates a grid-like pattern across a larger area of the retina.

photodynamic therapy—A newer treatment for AMD that involves the intravenous administration of a special drug to sensitize blood vessels in the eye to light. A low-power laser, directed at the new blood vessels, activates the drug and closes the vessels in a way that causes less damage to the retina than standard laser treatment.

posterior subcapsular cataract—A cataract in the rear of the lens capsule.

presbyopia—An inability to focus on near objects that commonly develops after age 45.

PRK—This stands for photorefractive keratotomy, a refractive surgery procedure that reshapes the cornea.

pupil—The opening in the center of the iris that resembles a large black dot.

retina—The innermost layer of the eye that consists of light-sensitive nerve tissue.

retinal detachment—A vision-threatening condition in which the retina becomes separated from the underlying layers of the eye.

retinal pigment epithelial cells—A layer of cells that contribute to the function of the retina.

rods—Nerve cells in the retina that are sensitive to dim light.

rubeosis iridis—New blood vessel growth on the iris that usually occurs in people with diabetes.

sclera—The white outer layer that covers and protects most of the eye.

scotoma—A blind spot in the visual field.

shunt—A device that creates a new passage to drain excess aqueous humor. It is used in the treatment of glaucoma when filtration surgery is unsuccessful.

slit lamp—A table-mounted microscope that enables an eye specialist to get a 3-dimensional view of the optic nerve.

subfoveal blood vessels—See neovascular AMD.

subfoveal surgery—A procedure for age-related macular degeneration in which abnormal blood vessels beneath the retina are surgically removed.

tonometry—A method of measuring intraocular pressure by determining the amount of force needed to make a slight indentation in a small area of the cornea.

topical prostaglandin eyedrops—A treatment for glaucoma. These eyedrops reduce intraocular pressure by increasing the outflow of aqueous humor through the uveoscleral pathway.

trabecular meshwork—A spongy network of connective tissue through which aqueous humor drains from the eye. Blockage of the meshwork causes a buildup of intraocular pressure.

trabeculectomy—See filtration surgery.

uveitis—Inflammation of the uvea, the part of the eye that contains the iris, ciliary body, and choroid.

uveoscleral pathway—An alternative drainage system for aqueous humor located behind the trabecular meshwork.

vascular endothelial growth factor (VEGF)—A protein that promotes the growth of new blood vessels in the eye and elsewhere in the body.

verteporfin—A drug used in photodynamic therapy and sold under the name of Visudyne.

vitrectomy—A surgical procedure that removes the vitreous humor and replaces it with saline solution.

vitreous humor—A thick, gel-like substance that fills the back of the eyeball behind the lens.

wet AMD—See neovascular AMD.

YAG laser—A type of laser that contains yttrium, aluminum, and garnet used to clear blurred vision that may occur after extracapsular surgery for cataracts.

HEALTH INFORMATION ORGANIZATIONS AND SUPPORT GROUPS

American Academy of Ophthalmology
P.O. Box 7424
San Francisco, CA 94120-7424
☎ 415-561-8500
www.aao.org
Largest association of ophthalmologists in the United States, with more than 27,000 members. For information on a variety of eye-related diseases and their prevention and treatment, describe your ailment(s) and send a self-addressed, stamped business envelope.

American Council of the Blind
1155 15th St. NW, Ste. 1004
Washington, DC 20005
☎ 800-424-8666/202-467-5081
www.acb.org
National information clearinghouse that also offers group insurance plans and other services.

American Optometric Association
243 North Lindbergh Blvd.
St. Louis, MO 63141
☎ 800-365-2219
www.aoanet.org
A professional group of doctors of optometry that lobbies the government and other organizations on behalf of the optometric profession, provides research and education leadership, and sets professional standards, helping its members conduct patient care efficiently and effectively.

Association for Macular Diseases, Inc.
210 East 64th St.
New York, NY 10021
☎ 212-605-3719
www.macula.org/association/about.html
Not-for-profit corporation devoted solely to macular disease. Membership includes a support group and a newsletter devoted to medical advances, new developments in low vision aids, and advice on coping strategies.

The Foundation Fighting Blindness
11435 Cronhill Dr.
Owings Mills, MD 21117-2220
☎ 800-394-3937
800-683-5555(TDD)
www.blindness.org
Supports research and provides education about retinal degeneration. Publishes a newsletter titled *Fighting Blindness News.*

Glaucoma Research Foundation
251 Post St., Ste. 600
San Francisco, CA 94108
☎ 800-826-6693/415-986-3162
www.glaucoma.org
National nonprofit organization committed to protecting the sight of people with glaucoma through research and education. Call the toll-free number for free publications.

Lighthouse International
111 E. 59th St.
New York, NY 10022
☎ 800-829-0500/212-821-9200
www.lighthouse.org
National nonprofit vision rehabilitation organization that conducts research and offers educational opportunities and direct services for people with vision loss.

National Association for the Visually Handicapped
22 W. 21st St., 6th Fl.
New York, NY 10010
☎ 212-889-3141/212-255-2804
www.navh.org
Volunteer health agency dedicated to serving the partially seeing. Publishes a quarterly large-print newsletter, medical updates, and other publications. Services include sale and/or referral of currently available vision aids and an extensive free-by-mail library of large-print books.

National Eye Institute Information Office
2020 Vision Place
Bethesda, MD 20892-3655
☎ 800-869-2020 (for publications)
301-496-5248 (public inquiry)
www.nei.nih.gov
Part of the National Institutes of Health. Provides information packets on a variety of eye ailments and answers inquiries over the phone. Supports more than 75% of the vision research conducted in the United States.

Prevent Blindness America
211 West Wacker Drive, Ste. 1700
Chicago, IL 60606
☎ 800-331-2020
www.preventblindness.org
Provides public and professional education, vision screenings, community programs, toll-free hotline, and research.

Vision World Wide, Inc.
5707 Brockton Dr., #302
Indianapolis, IN 46220-5481
☎ 800-431-1739/317-254-1332
www.visionww.org
Provides publications in large print, on audiocassette, on computer disk, or in electronic format (PDF or ASCII text). Call the toll-free number for information and referral services.

LEADING HOSPITALS FOR OPHTHALMOLOGY

U.S. News & World Report and the National Opinion Research Center, a social-science research group at the University of Chicago, recently conducted their 16th annual nationwide survey of 3,400 board-certified physicians in 17 medical specialties. The doctors nominated the hospitals that they considered to be the best from among 6,007 U.S. medical centers.

This is the current list of the best hospitals for ophthalmology, as determined by doctors' recommendations from 2003, 2004, and 2005. However, because the results reflect the doctors' opinions, they are subjective. Any institution listed is considered a leading center, and the rankings do not imply that other hospitals cannot or do not deliver excellent care.

1. **University of Miami (Bascom Palmer Eye Institute)**
   Miami, FL
   ☎ 305-243-2020
   www.bpei.med.miami.edu

2. **Johns Hopkins Hospital (Wilmer Eye Institute)**
   Baltimore, MD
   ☎ 410-955-5080
   www.wilmer.jhu.edu

3. **Wills Eye Hospital**
   Philadelphia, PA
   ☎ 215-928-3000
   www.willseye.org

4. **Massachusetts Eye and Ear Infirmary**
   Boston, MA
   ☎ 617-523-7900
   www.meei.harvard.edu

5. **University of California, Los Angeles, Medical Center (Jules Stein Eye Institute)**
   Los Angeles, CA
   ☎ 310-825-5000
   www.jsei.org

6. **University of Iowa Hospitals and Clinics**
   Iowa City, IA
   ☎ 800-777-8442/319-384-8442
   www.uihealthcare.com/uihospitalsandclinics

7. **University of Southern California University Hospital (Doheny Eye Institute)**
   Los Angeles, CA
   ☎ 323-442-6335
   www.usc.edu/hsc/doheny

8. **Duke University Medical Center**
   Durham, NC
   ☎ 919-684-8111
   www.dukehealth.org

9. **Barnes-Jewish Hospital**
   St. Louis, MO
   ☎ 314-747-3000
   www.barnesjewish.org

10. **Mayo Clinic**
    Rochester, MN
    ☎ 507-284-2511
    www.mayoclinic.org

JOHNS HOPKINS
MEDICINE

THE JOHNS HOPKINS WHITE PAPERS

Selected Medical Journal Article

MILESTONES IN AGE-RELATED MACULAR DEGENERATION RESEARCH

The advanced stages of age-related macular degeneration (AMD) are currently estimated to affect more than 1.75 million people in the United States. Based on demographic projections, that number will increase by 50% to nearly 3 million people in less than 20 years.

Most current treatments are limited to the advanced stages of AMD, when central vision is already under great threat. Thus, the race is on to find treatments for earlier stages and, ideally, effective strategies for prevention.

Stuart L. Fine, MD, the author of the review article reprinted on the following pages, has been at the forefront of AMD research during his career. In this article, which reflects his personal experience in treating patients with AMD and his collegial relationships with other leading researchers, Dr. Fine provides a chronological overview of the important milestones in AMD research since 1969 and identifies some promising areas for future research.

During the past 35 years, as Dr. Fine notes, researchers have come a long way in terms of identifying important risk factors and developing new treatments for AMD. While year-to-year research results may seem to offer only incremental steps forward, the broad picture provides another story. AMD treatment today is substantially different than it was even 10 years ago, much less 35 years ago. Indeed, as Dr. Fine puts it, AMD has moved from the rear balcony to center stage.

Age-Related Macular Degeneration 1969–2004: A 35-Year Personal Perspective

STUART L. FINE, MD

• PURPOSE: To provide a personal perspective concerning diagnosis, treatment, and evaluation of treatment for early and late stages of age-related macular degeneration (AMD) over a 35 year period, 1969–2004.
• DESIGN: Literature review, personal recollections, and conversations with investigators who participated in trials to evaluate treatments for AMD.
• METHODS: The author reviewed the literature pertaining to evaluation and treatment of patients with AMD and conversed with investigators who, over the past 35 years, designed, conducted and participated in trials to assess new and existing treatments for AMD.
• RESULTS: In 1969, patients with AMD constituted a small part of a typical ophthalmic practice. From 1969 to 2004, the prevalence of AMD has increased, and the methods of evaluation and treatment have changed dramatically. The emergence of fluorescein angiography and the development of laser photocoagulation and photodynamic therapy have substantially altered clinical practice. Several promising pharmacologic interventions are now being assessed in clinical trials. Nevertheless, AMD remains the leading cause of severe and irreversible vision loss in the United States because there are no highly effective treatments available for most patients.
• CONCLUSIONS: Because of an aging population and the lack of highly effective treatments, late AMD remains a major unsolved problem. However, there is extensive research being conducted with support from the National Eye Institute and from industry. There is also great interest in prevention trials. Accordingly, the author is optimistic that over the next 35 years there will be significant improvements in our ability to prevent severe vision loss from late AMD. (Am J Ophthalmol 2005;139:405–420. © 2005 by Elsevier Inc. All rights reserved.)

Accepted for publication Nov 18, 2004.
From the Scheie Eye Institute, Department of Ophthalmology, University of Pennsylvania, Philadelphia, Pennsylvania.
Supported, in part, by Research to Prevent Blindness, Inc., New York, New York, National Eye Institute grant No. U10-EY-012261, (Complications of AMD Prevention Trial), the Paul Mackall and Evanina Evans Bell Mackall Trust, the Scheie Eye Institute Macular Degeneration Research Fund, the F.M. Kirby Foundation, and the Rosanne Silbermann Foundation.
Inquiries to Stuart L. Fine, MD, University of Pennsylvania, 51 North 39th Street, Philadelphia, PA 19104; fax: 215-662-9676; e-mail: stuart.fine@uphs.upenn.edu

THIS PRESENTATION IS A HISTORICAL PERSPECTIVE on the development of risk factor data and on the evolution of treatments for macular degeneration which have guided patient care since I began my residency in 1969. As depicted in Table 1, the presentation is divided into four eras that coincide with what I consider important milestones.

This retrospective begins in the early 1960s with the advent of fluorescein fundus photography, an innovation which facilitated Gass's seminal 1967 publications demonstrating that leakage from abnormal choroidal vessels was responsible for the exudative manifestations in age-related macular degeneration (AMD).[1] In the early 1970s, few centers were equipped to perform fluorescein fundus photography, and the quality of the angiograms was generally poor. Apart from low vision aids, the most popular treatment was a multivitamin. While there were occasional reports about photocoagulation, there was no agreed upon protocol for performing or evaluating laser treatment.

Figure 1 summarizes the understanding in the 1970s about the pathogenesis of choroidal neovascularization (CNV), specifically, that a break in Bruch's membrane permitted choroidal blood vessels to penetrate and leak into the sub-retinal pigment epithelial (RPE) space. There was no mention of growth factors or other angiogenic stimuli.

There was correspondingly little information with regard to AMD risk factors, apart from age and family history. The Framingham Eye Study monograph, published in 1980, first identified AMD as a major cause of blindness in the United States.[2] Even the name was different. Until the mid-1980s, the condition was called by the pejorative and medically inappropriate "senile macular degeneration," a term which had been used for more than 100 years.

With regard to risk factors, the role of genetics, smoking, cardiovascular disease, dietary history, sunlight exposure, and other possible risk factors would be studied and reported on during the next decade by a number of investigative groups led by Drs. Leslie Hyman at the Johns Hopkins School of Hygiene and Public Health,[3] Bressler NM, Bressler SB, West S, et al. from the Chesapeake Bay Watermen Study,[4] Barbara and Ron Klein from the Beaver Dam Eye Study,[5–8] Paul Mitchell from the Blue Mountains

REPRINT

TABLE 1. Four Eras Representing Milestones in the Development of Risk Factor Data and in Evolution of Treatments for AMD, 1969–2004

1st Era: 1969–1979
- Emergence of fluorescein fundus photography
- Development of argon laser photocoagulation
- Relationship of drusen to age-related macular degeneration

2nd Era: 1979–1994
- Clinical trials to evaluate new treatments, especially laser photocoagulation
- Development of risk factor data from large and small epidemiologic studies

3rd Era: 1994–2004
- Evaluation of radiation therapy for neovascular AMD
- Assessment of pharmacologic interventions for neovascular AMD
- Prevention trials

4th Era: 2004 -
- Completion of ongoing trials for neovascular AMD
- Earlier identification of eyes at risk
- Prevention trials in pre-symptomatic patients

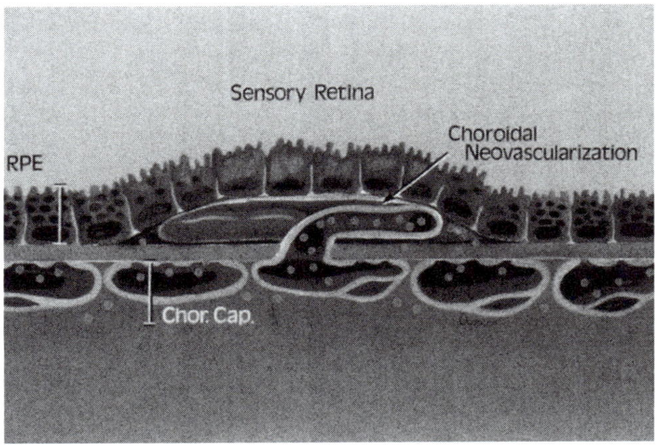

FIGURE 1. 1970s sketch illustrating break in Bruch's membrane as underlying feature leading to the development of choroidal neovascularization.

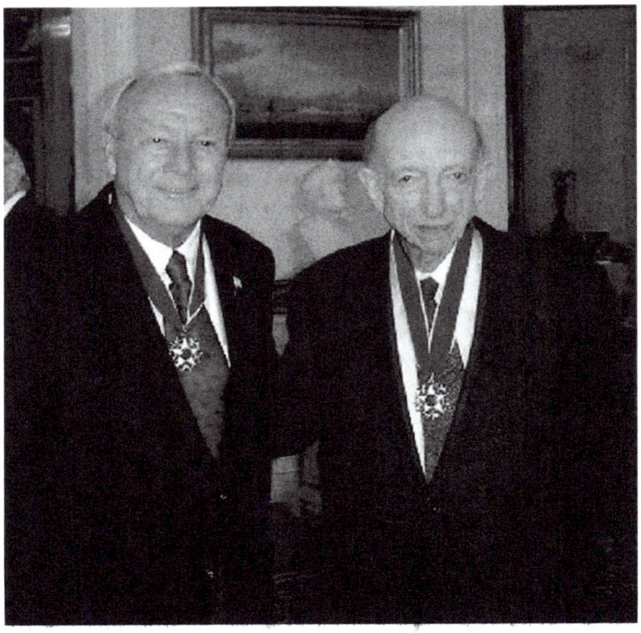

FIGURE 2. Arnall Patz (right) and Arnold Palmer (left). Patz received the Presidential Medal of Freedom at the White House in June 2004 for establishing the relationship between oxygen and retinopathy of prematurity in low birth weight infants.

Eye Study,[9] Paulus de Jong from the Rotterdam Study,[10,11] investigators participating in the NEI-sponsored Eye Disease Case Control Study,[12,13] and many others.[14–16]

In the 1970s, it would have been unusual for the AAO annual meeting program to have included symposia, courses, posters, or exhibits devoted to AMD. Then, in 1976, a major breakthrough occurred. The April 1976 issue of the American Journal of Ophthalmology described the benefits of panretinal photocoagulation or PRP in the treatment of proliferative and severe non-proliferative diabetic retinopathy.[17] In addition to documenting the substantial benefits of PRP, the 1976 DRS report provided a second lesson of equal importance. It demonstrated the power of the randomized clinical trial in the assessment of new treatments, especially for problems of major public health importance. Nearly 25 years had elapsed since the landmark publications by Arnall Patz et al. which documented that high oxygen in low birth weight premature infants increased the incidence of retrolental fibroplasia (RLF), the original name for retinopathy of prematurity, contributions recognized at the time by the Albert and Mary Lasker Award and most recently by the Presidential Medal of Freedom awarded to Dr. Patz. (Figure 2).[18,19] Edward Jackson, the educator (Figure 3), would have been interested to know that PRP, the most effective treatment introduced into any area of medicine over the past 30 years, except for vaccines, was preceded by a period in which those who developed the treatment technique were often ridiculed for proposing that a treatment which ablated one quarter or more of the retina actually might be helpful! Patz had encountered similar skepticism in the 1950s when he proposed that high oxygen might contribute to the incidence of RLF.

The 1976 DRS publication ushered in the next era, 1979–1994, during which time three randomized trials were conducted to evaluate laser treatment for neovascular AMD. The trials were led by Bird, Chisholm, and colleagues at Moorfields Eye Hospital in London,[20] by Coscas and Soubrane at the University of Creteil in France,[21] and by the Macular Photocoagulation Study (MPS) group at 16 centers in the United States.[22] In 1982, all three groups reported that laser photocoagulation, when employed to treat choroidal neovascularization outside the fovea, reduced the risk of severe vision loss compared to observa-

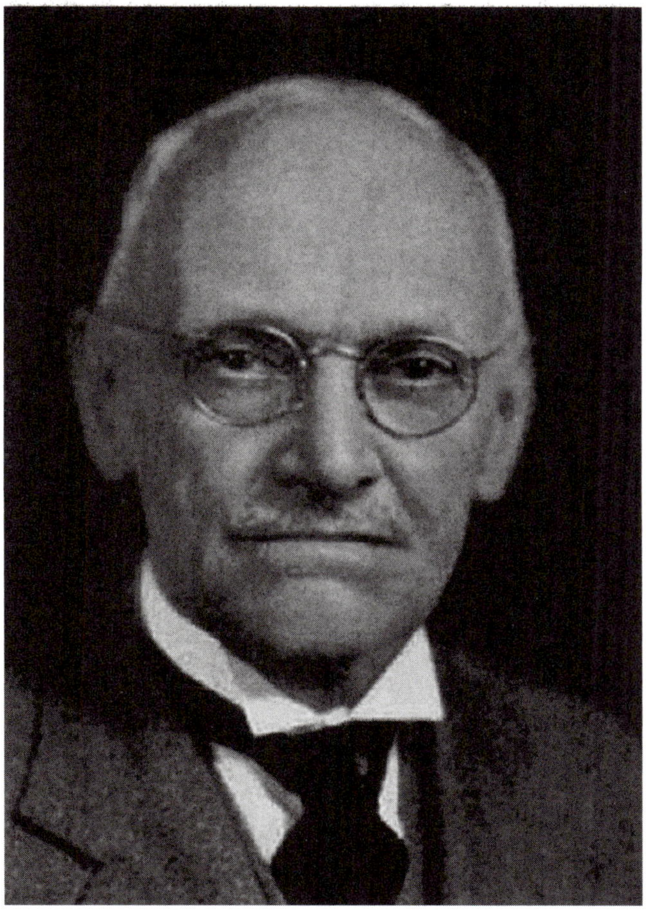

FIGURE 3. Edward Jackson (1856–1942).

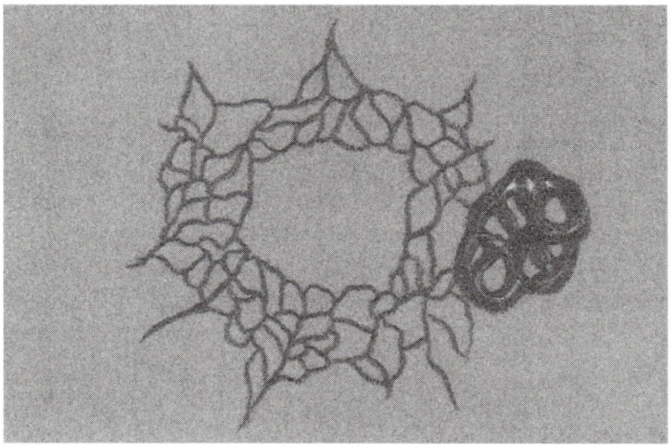

FIGURE 4. Sketch illustrates well-defined choroidal neovascularization outside the fovea. Neovascular lesions in this location were shown to benefit from treatment with laser photocoagulation.

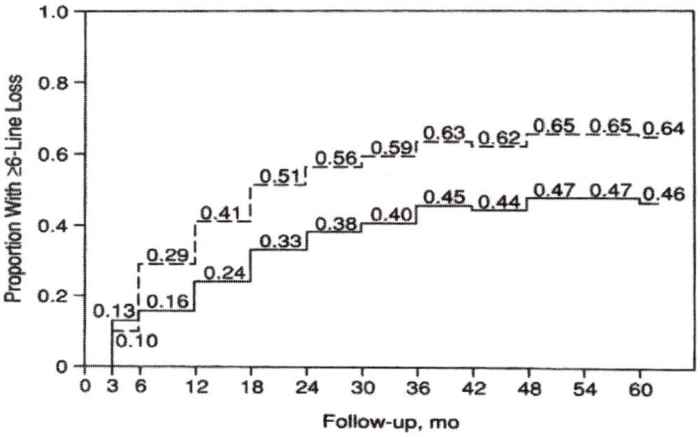

FIGURE 5. Reprinted with permission from Archives of Ophthalmology, Vol 100, p. 916, June 1982, "Cumulative Proportion of Eyes With Event (in MPS Trial of argon laser photocoagulation for extrafoveal choroidal neovascularization). Event has been defined as decrease in visual acuity of six or more lines from baseline. Dashed line indicates no treatment group; solid line, treatment group."

tion (Figure 4).[20–22] The 60-month visual outcome data from the MPS are shown in Figure 5.

Despite these favorable reports from three well conducted clinical trials, there are two major limitations to laser treatment for CNV in patients with AMD: (1) Only a small proportion of patients with neovascular AMD is eligible for laser treatment by virtue of having a fluorescein angiographically well defined area of leakage outside the fovea; and (2) There is a high rate of recurrent leakage after initial laser treatment. Notwithstanding these limitations, laser has remained the treatment of choice for patients with extrafoveal new vessels for more than 20 years. One measure of its value is that, in MPS laser-treated eyes that did not develop recurrent leakage, the average visual acuity three years after treatment was 20/50. In comparison, in laser-treated eyes that did develop recurrent leakage, the average visual acuity three years after treatment was 20/250.[23]

It is interesting to recall that when these three laser trials were conducted, choroidal neovascularization was diagnosed with certainty only when it had angiographic features of what we now call classic CNV (Figure 6). Although areas of abnormal fluorescence adjacent to classic CNV were considered to represent a variant of neovascularization, the term occult CNV was not yet part of our clinical vocabulary (Figure 7). It would be several years before occult CNV would be acknowledged as the predominant form of neovascularization in patients with AMD.

In my role as MPS Chair, I recall two vignettes of interest. First, the grant proposal to the National Eye Institute requesting support to conduct a trial of laser treatment for neovascular AMD was initially disapproved for funding by a study section. The summary statement from the review stated that laser photocoagulation actually caused choroidal neovascularization and therefore could not be considered as a treatment for choroidal neovascularization. This conclusion was based on erroneous extrap-

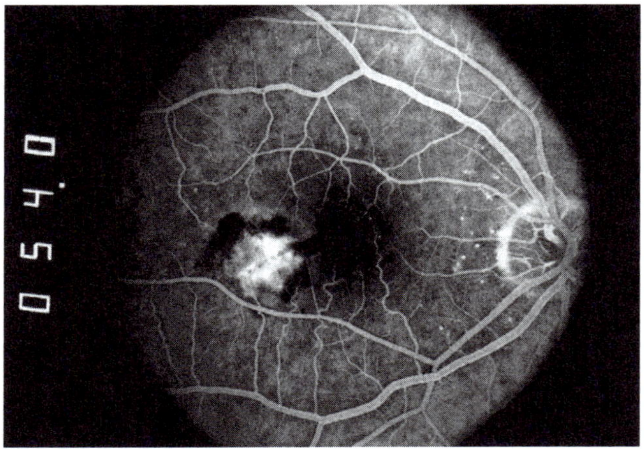

FIGURE 6. Treatment of choroidal neovascularization in 1970s. Fluorescein angiogram shows well defined area of choroidal neovascularization not involving the foveal avascular zone.

olation from two publications. The first article, by Schatz et al., described several patients diagnosed with central serous chorioretinopathy and treated with argon laser photocoagulation who, shortly after laser treatment, were discovered to have choroidal neovascularization, purportedly as a complication of the laser treatment.[24] The second article was a publication by Ryan on the now well known monkey model for producing choroidal neovascularization in primates by delivering short bursts of high intensity laser application to rupture Bruch's membrane, thereby facilitating the emergence of choroidal new vessels.[25] My co-investigators and I thought that the study section's conclusions, based on their extrapolations from these two publications, were flawed because, in both these articles, the laser parameters were small diameter laser burns of short duration delivered at moderate to high energy, whereas our laser treatment protocol was proposing larger diameter burns of longer duration. Accordingly, we appealed to the National Advisory Eye Council to support our proposal based not only on the flawed review but also on the public health importance of age-related macular degeneration. Fortunately, the Council agreed with our reasoning, and the Macular Photocoagulation Study was funded beginning in 1978.

The second vignette from the MPS provided an invaluable and never forgotten lesson. Patient enrollment for the MPS began in 1979. A Data and Safety Monitoring Committee appointed by NEI Director, Carl Kupfer, reviewed the accumulating data at six-month intervals. In January 1982, with 224 patients enrolled, this committee noted that, after 18 months of follow up, 60% of untreated eyes compared to only 25% of laser-treated eyes had experienced six or more lines of visual acuity loss. Based on those outcome data, the DSMC voted unanimously to recommend that study enrollment be halted; that all investigators, study patients, and the ophthalmic community be informed; and that all study patients be evaluated to determine their eligibility for laser treatment.

It in was my charge to arrange a meeting of the 16 MPS principal investigators so that the DSMC Chair could present the findings. I was asked not to reveal the outcome data but only to schedule the meeting so that study results could be presented. During telephone conversations, I could not resist asking investigators, all experienced retina specialists, whether they thought the outcome would be in favor of laser or observation. Of the 15 retina specialists representing the other clinical centers, all but one opined that laser treatment probably was not helpful! That response provided a lesson never forgotten, namely, that even experienced clinicians can reach erroneous conclusions based on following a few dozen patients without an appropriate comparison group.

The initial MPS outcome data were presented at a national press conference arranged by the National Eye Institute and convened at the National Institutes of Health in Bethesda in May 1982. The data were reported in an expedited publication in the Archives of Ophthalmology in June 1982.[22] The press conference received national attention from the three major television networks as well as from the New York Times, the Wall Street Journal, and print and broadcast media across the United States. Although efforts were made to inform the ophthalmic community about these findings by means of a prepublication manuscript mailed to all ophthalmologists in the United States in advance of the press conference, a number of practitioners heard about the MPS findings on the evening news before they had a chance to read the manuscript. Understandably, many patients called their ophthalmologists, asking about laser treatment, despite having had vision loss for years attributable to macular disciform scars, glaucoma, and other irreversible conditions.

Since the treatment benefit of argon laser for neovascular AMD was reported during approximately the same time period by investigators in the United Kingdom,[20] France,[21] and the United States,[22] the retina communities on both sides of the Atlantic and around the world quickly adopted recommendations for treating patients with CNV outside the fovea. In the weeks and months following the 1982 publications, large numbers of patients, including all MPS participants who had been assigned to the observation group, were evaluated to determine their eligibility for laser treatment. Unfortunately, only a small proportion of patients with neovascular maculopathy secondary to AMD actually have well defined extrafoveal choroidal neovascularization. Thus, there was understandably a great deal of frustration among patients and their ophthalmologists.

During the 1979–1994 era, many investigators around the globe contributed data, provided insights, and developed or applied technology to assist with diagnosis and study design. Among these contributions are those by Flower, Yannuzzi, and Guyer on ICG angiography,[26] Pu-

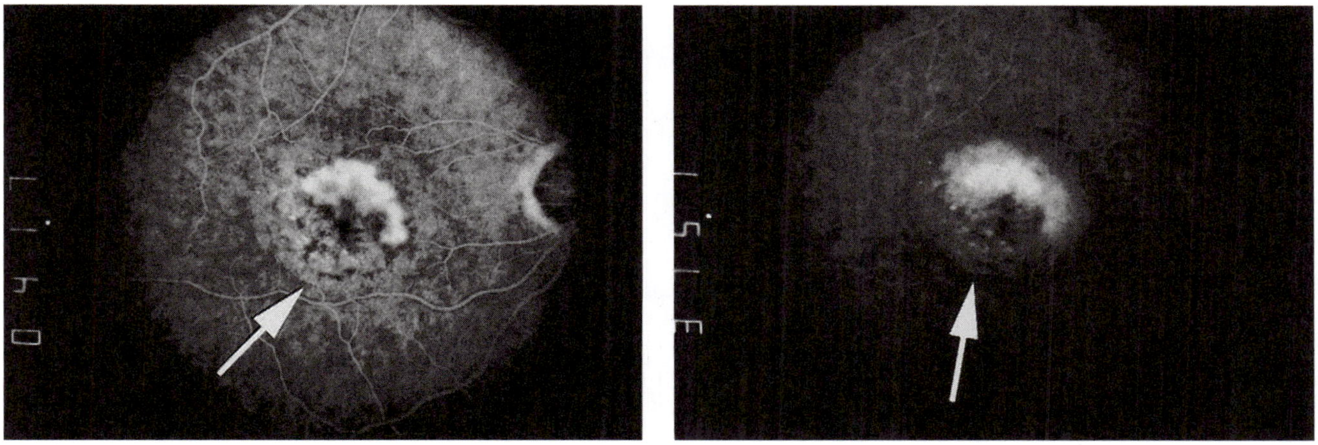

FIGURE 7. Fluorescein angiogram shows area of classic choroidal neovascularization with adjacent area of abnormal fluorescence (arrow) now recognized as occult CNV. (A) Early phase angiogram. (B) Late phase angiogram.

liafito and colleagues on optical coherence tomography,[27] Bird and the International Classification of AMD Group,[28] the MPS investigators on classification of choroidal neovascularization,[29] and many others. Never to be forgotten or taken for granted are the patients who volunteered as subjects for these studies.

The years between 1979 and 1994 also witnessed the emergence of important risk factor data beginning with the 1980 Framingham Eye Study monograph and continuing with information from many population-based epidemiologic studies whose principal authors already have been acknowledged. In my corner of the world, colleagues who at the time were medical students, and I conducted risk factor studies on several categories of AMD patients.

- Susan and Neil Bressler reported that, among untreated eyes with juxtafoveal neovascularization, 89% had visual acuity of 20/200 or worse within 24 months.[30]
- David Guyer reported that 64% of eyes with untreated subfoveal neovascularization lost 6 or more lines of vision within 24 months.[31]

These natural history data provided impetus for the MPS investigators to assess laser treatment for juxtafoveal and subfoveal neovascularization in trials supported by the National Eye Institute. These trials concluded that laser treatment, compared to observation, reduced the risk of severe vision loss. In the trial evaluating krypton red laser treatment for juxtafoveal neovascular lesions (496 eyes in 494 patients), treatment reduced the risk of severe vision loss compared to observation when comparing all treated eyes with all untreated eyes.[32] The treatment benefit was particularly strong in normotensive patients and of no demonstrable benefit in hypertensive patients.[33]

The trial evaluating laser treatment for subfoveal neovascular lesions, known as the Foveal Photocoagulation Study (FPS), enrolled 373 eyes in 371 patients in the new subfoveal membrane study and 209 eyes in 209 patients in the recurrent subfoveal membrane study. In the trial of recurrent-subfoveal neovascular lesions (Figure 8), laser treatment proved to have a significant advantage over observation in terms of reducing the risk of severe vision loss. After two years, 8% of laser-treated eyes compared to 29% of observed eyes experienced severe vision loss.[34] Moreover, this treatment benefit was obtained irrespective of the size of the recurrent neovascularization as long as the eye met all the eligibility criteria for enrollment; for example, lesions could be no greater than six disk areas in extent, including the area of prior laser photocoagulation.

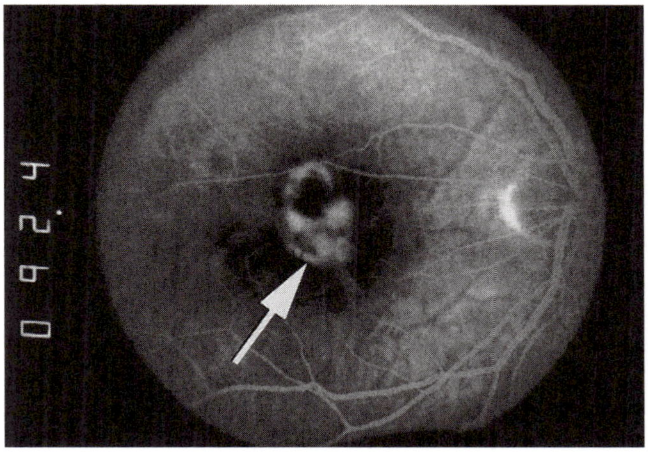

FIGURE 8. Fluorescein angiogram shows marginal recurrent leakage under the fovea (arrow) in eye previously treated with laser for extrafoveal choroidal neovascularization.

In the trial evaluating laser photocoagulation for new (previously untreated) subfoveal lesions, eyes which began with smaller neovascular lesions and worse visual acuity derived the greatest benefit from laser treatment. The benefit typically was a reduction in the rate of progression to severe vision loss.[35,36] In almost all cases, however,

TABLE 2. Risk Factors for Progression From Drusen to Choroidal Neovascularization in the Second (Fellow) Eyes of Patients with CNV in the First Eye

- Drusen number (>10)
- Drusen size (>125)
- Macular pigment clumping
- Systemic hypertension

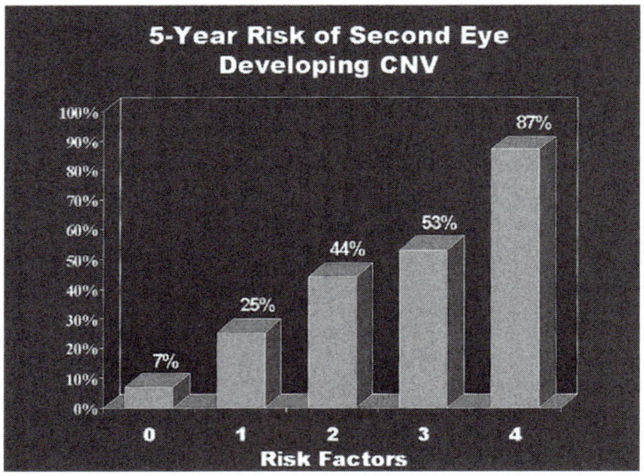

FIGURE 9. Five year risk of developing CNV in the second eye as a function of the number of risk factors present. (See Table 2 and Reference 38).

especially in patients with subfoveal neovascular lesions, laser treatment caused an immediate and usually irreversible decrease in central vision, an outcome not appreciated by patients or by their ophthalmologists. These trials, while successful with regard to design, conduct, completion, data analysis, and demonstration of a laser treatment benefit, provided additional impetus to search for less destructive treatments for AMD patients with subfoveal neovascularization.

In the 1980s, medical students with whom I collaborated also conducted studies which quantified the risk of progressing from drusen to neovascularization. Ellen Strahlman et al. identified drusen number, drusen size, and macular pigment clumping as risk factors for progression from drusen to CNV in fellow eyes of patients who already had developed CNV in their first eye.[37] These observations were subsequently confirmed and quantified among the MPS patient cohort with second eyes at risk.[38] The MPS also documented that systemic hypertension was an independent risk factor for progression from drusen to CNV (Table 2). The magnitude of this risk varies substantially according to the number of risk factors, information of great import in identifying patients with fellow eyes at greatest risk of vision loss who might be candidates for prevention trials (Figure 9).

In patients with drusen and good visual acuity in both eyes, Smiddy et al. and Holz et al. at Moorfields, independently reported that drusen number, drusen size, and macular pigment clumping were risk factors for progression to vision loss or choroidal neovascularization or both.[39,40] These risk factor data were useful in designing the Age-Related Eye Diseases Study (AREDS) by identifying patients at greatest risk of progression from drusen and good visual acuity to advanced AMD or vision loss.

The next era, which extends from 1994 to 2004, is characterized by pharmacologic intervention trials, radiotherapy trials, and prevention trials. The first trial evaluated oral thalidomide in patients with subfoveal neovascularization. The rationale for this trial was based on experiments conducted by Robert D'Amato, MD, PhD. After completing a residency at the Massachusetts Eye and Ear Infirmary, D'Amato was mentored by Dr. Judah Folkman at Children's Hospital Boston. For several decades, an important objective for the Folkman laboratory had been to discover or develop drugs that would inhibit angiogenesis in patients with cancer. This objective was based on the assumption that solid tumors deprived of a blood supply would be less likely to grow. Both Folkman and D'Amato recognized the similarities between tumor angiogenesis and ocular angiogenesis. During a comprehensive literature review to identify drugs that might have anti-angiogenic activity, D'Amato encountered thalidomide, a drug that inhibited menstruation and caused birth defects. Since 1963, the sale of thalidomide had been banned because of its teratogenic effect on fetal development if taken by pregnant women during the first trimester. After a literature review, D'Amato concluded that thalidomide crossed the placental barrier and inhibited blood vessel growth in the limbs of the developing fetus. He reasoned that it would likely cross the blood-brain and blood-ocular barriers as well.

To test the hypothesis that thalidomide might be an effective angio-inhibitory drug in the eye, D'Amato performed experiments in rabbits in which pellets impregnated with basic fibroblast growth factor (bFGF) were placed in a central corneal pocket to induce ingrowth of vessels from the corneal limbus. Rabbits treated with thalidomide experienced a 65% reduction in corneal neovascularization compared to controls (Figure 10).[41] These experiments, which confirmed the angio-inhibitory properties of thalidomide, also explained the dysmelia that occurred in infants whose mothers had taken thalidomide during the first trimester of pregnancy; specifically, if angiogenesis in the limb is inhibited, the limb does not develop properly.

During the 1994 ARVO meeting, D'Amato described to me the results of the thalidomide experiments using the rabbit cornea model. I learned at that time that thalidomide had been used for many years as an effective treatment for patients with leprosy, severe rheumatoid arthritis, and for some patients with graft vs host disease. In each of these conditions, the drug was reported to be well tolerated with only minimal side effects consisting of drowsiness, constipation, and a largely reversible peripheral neuropathy which reportedly occurred in approxi-

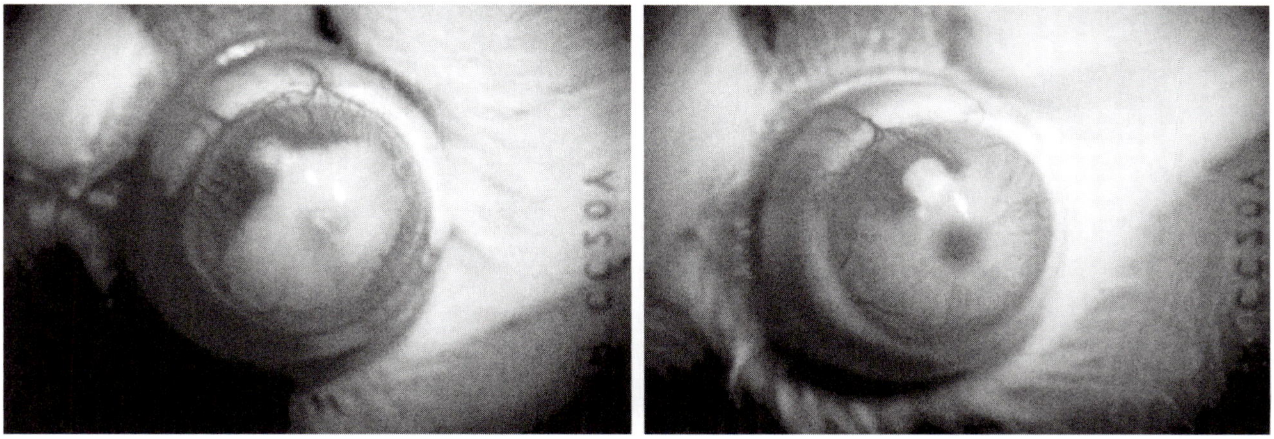

FIGURE 10. Rabbit corneas eight days after implantation of bFGF pellets in central corneal pocket. (A) Control. (B) Thalidomide-treated. (Photographs courtesy of Robert D'Amato, MD, PhD, Harvard Medical School, Children's Hospital of Boston.)

mately 5% of treated patients. In view of these data and in recognition of the urgent need for a more effective treatment for AMD patients with subfoveal neovascularization, it seemed appropriate to evaluate thalidomide for patients with subfoveal CNV. The reported side effects seemed manageable, and the issue of fetal toxicity would be non-existent since the average age of patients with neovascular AMD was 70 to 75 years.

Thus, with approval of a protocol by the FDA, my colleagues and I began a trial of low dose thalidomide in AMD patients with subfoveal neovascular lesions. However, only 22% of 18 patients assigned to thalidomide continued their medication throughout 12 months compared to 65% of 20 patients assigned to the placebo group. The trial could not be completed as designed because the peripheral neuropathy and other side effects proved to be considerably more frequent and more disabling than previously reported, despite the fact that the patients started with a low dose (150 mg) at bedtime and increased to 150 mg twice daily if the initial dose was well tolerated. The conclusion from the AMD Thalidomide Study was that, because of the disabling side effects, thalidomide could not be considered as a treatment for patients with neovascular AMD (unpublished data).

The 1990s witnessed the completion of two concurrent multicenter trials conducted worldwide to evaluate interferon alfa-2a as a treatment for AMD patients with subfoveal CNV. These trials were conducted after a relatively small number of patients who had been treated with interferon appeared to improve more often than historical controls. The two multicenter trials showed that interferon, when administered according to study protocol, was not an effective treatment for neovascular AMD.[42] In one sub-group, interferon-treated patients actually experienced a worse visual outcome than observed patients.

The 1994–2004 decade also witnessed the conduct of several radiotherapy trials. In the United Kingdom, Chakravarthy and colleagues had demonstrated that radiation impaired proliferation of vascular endothelial cells.[43] Two well conducted trials, one in the U.K. and one in Germany, failed to show that low dose radiation was an effective treatment.[44,45] The German collaborative trial, which involved nine centers, concluded that 16 Gy of radiation therapy, administered in 8 doses of 2 Gy each, was not beneficial in preventing vision loss among AMD patients with subfoveal CNV.[45] A point to emphasize is that this well conducted trial could draw a conclusion only about the radiation dose that was evaluated.[46]

Another group of investigators chose to evaluate a dose of 20 Gy of external beam radiation therapy administered as 5 divided doses of 4 Gy each, in a similar group of AMD patients with subfoveal CNV. This AMD Radiotherapy Trial (AMDRT), supported by the National Eye Institute, found that after six months of follow up, 26% of radiation-treated eyes compared to 50% of eyes not radiated, lost $\geq$3 lines of visual acuity (P = .04). At 12 months, 43% of radiated and 50% of observed eyes lost $\geq$3 lines of visual acuity (P = .60). Also at 12 months, the radiation-treated group demonstrated smaller lesions and less fibrosis than the observed group (P = .05 and .004 respectively).[47] Although this dose of radiation may have a modest treatment benefit of short duration, the treatment benefit is not overwhelming, thus it seems unlikely at this time that radiotherapy will become a major therapeutic option for AMD patients with subfoveal CNV.

The mid-point of the 1994–2004 decade, 1999, marked the first of a series of publications on Verteporfin-Photodynamic Therapy (PDT) as treatment for neovascular AMD and related maculopathies.[48] The biologic basis of photodynamic therapy (PDT) is based on the interaction between a light absorbing chromophore which, when activated by a particular wavelength, leads to the initiation of a chemical reaction of therapeutic benefit. Some investigators who pioneered the application of photodynamic therapy to the treatment of choroidal neovascularization were Drs. Joan Miller, Evangelos Gragoudos, and Ursula

REPRINT

Schmidt-Erfurth who performed their basic research at the Wellpoint Photobiology Lab at Harvard and at the Massachusetts Eye and Ear Infirmary.[49] Their findings, which informed the clinical protocols, provided critical information concerning dosage of drug, duration of light exposure, frequency of treatment, and intervals between treatment. When the phase I/II trials showed that PDT with verteporfin (Novartis Pharma AG, Basel, Switzerland) could cause temporary cessation of fluorescein leakage from CNV, that recurring leakage could be halted with repeat application of PDT, and that intravenously injected verteporfin appeared to be safe, two large multicenter phase III trials were launched.[50]

The initial report from these trials documented that verteporfin photodynamic therapy was beneficial for patients with subfoveal choroidal neovascularization that had evidence of classic CNV. Subgroup analyses suggested that the benefit was mainly in those with a predominantly classic composition on fluorescein angiography. Subsequent reports have documented the benefit of PDT for eyes with occult with no classic choroidal neovascularization with recent disease progression and for eyes with relatively small, minimally classic choroidal neovascularization.[51] Ongoing analyses have shown that lesion size is an important factor in determining the efficacy of photodynamic therapy in patients with minimally classic or purely occult neovascularization.[52] Lesions less than four disk areas in extent have the most favorable prognosis.

In all the studies of PDT for choroidal neovascularization secondary to AMD, only individuals with subfoveal neovascular lesions were eligible for enrollment because thermal laser photocoagulation has remained the treatment of choice for patients with extrafoveal neovascular lesions. However, since only a minority of choroidal neovascular lesions in AMD is extrafoveal, photodynamic therapy has by default become the treatment of choice for the majority of AMD patients with CNV who might be considered for any form of treatment. As was the case after the benefits of thermal laser treatment were first documented in trials and adopted in clinical practice, both ophthalmologists and patients recognize the limitations of PDT and eagerly anticipate treatments for neovascular AMD that are more effective.

Several ongoing trials are evaluating drugs which inhibit angiogenesis. Treatment regimens currently under investigation include Retaane (Alcon, Fort Worth, Texas, USA), Lucentis (Genentech, South San Francisco, California, USA), and Macugen (Eyetech Pharmaceuticals, New York, New York, USA). Ongoing reports from these studies, as well as from continuing efforts to refine the role of PDT, with and without triamcinolone, will be featured presentations at meetings over the next 12 to 24 months. Future reports should place each of these treatments in perspective. If any of these interventions has a beneficial effect, it would seem incumbent to compare its advantages and limitations with existing treatments by means of a controlled trial.

Trials to evaluate prophylactic interventions evolved in the 1994–2004 era with the conduct of a micronutrient supplementation trial, two laser trials, and a pharmacologic intervention trial. The possibility of prophylaxis has been a most exciting development because an effective intervention for early AMD almost certainly would have a far greater impact on reducing vision loss than any intervention for late AMD.[53]

The first prevention trial was AREDS whose initial outcome data were published in 2001.[54] AREDS initially was conceived as a natural history study. Two considerations promoted its evolution to a trial. First was the recognition that many elderly patients already were taking micronutrient supplements based on marketing instead of evidence. Second was the notion that providing patients with a pill might bond the patients to a study with a prolonged follow-up period. After an average of 6.3 years of follow-up, the group of patients with large drusen in both eyes (AREDS Group 3) as well as the cohort of patients who already had experienced vision loss from late AMD in one eye and had a second eye at risk (AREDS Group 4), experienced a 20% relative reduction in the risk of three lines of vision loss and a 25% relative reduction in the risk of progressing to advanced AMD if they had been assigned to take the study formulation which included antioxidant vitamins, zinc, and copper (Figure 11). When patient enrollment began, not even the study leaders, Drs. Frederick Ferris and Emily Chew, could envision that micronutrients actually might have such a significant impact. Again we witness the power of the randomized trial to provide unassailable information that guides patient care, especially for important public health problems. Appropriately, the ophthalmic community has adopted the AREDS recommendations that patients with high risk drusen or unilateral advanced AMD benefit substantially by taking the formulation which includes antioxidant vitamins, zinc, and copper.

Two ongoing trials are evaluating whether low intensity laser photocoagulation can reduce progression from drusen to advanced AMD and vision loss. Efforts at prevention of disease progression in AMD using laser began as early as the 1970s when several investigators including Gass, Cleasby, Little, and Wetzig reported at various meetings that treating drusen directly with xenon arc, argon laser, or ruby laser photocoagulation, led to their partial or complete disappearance. All of these reports and presentations described relatively small numbers of patients with relatively short follow-up, and most suffered from the absence of controls achieved by means of randomization. If there were merit, anatomic or visual, to applying laser treatment as a preventive strategy in eyes with drusen, a large controlled clinical trial would be necessary to establish the benefit or lack thereof.

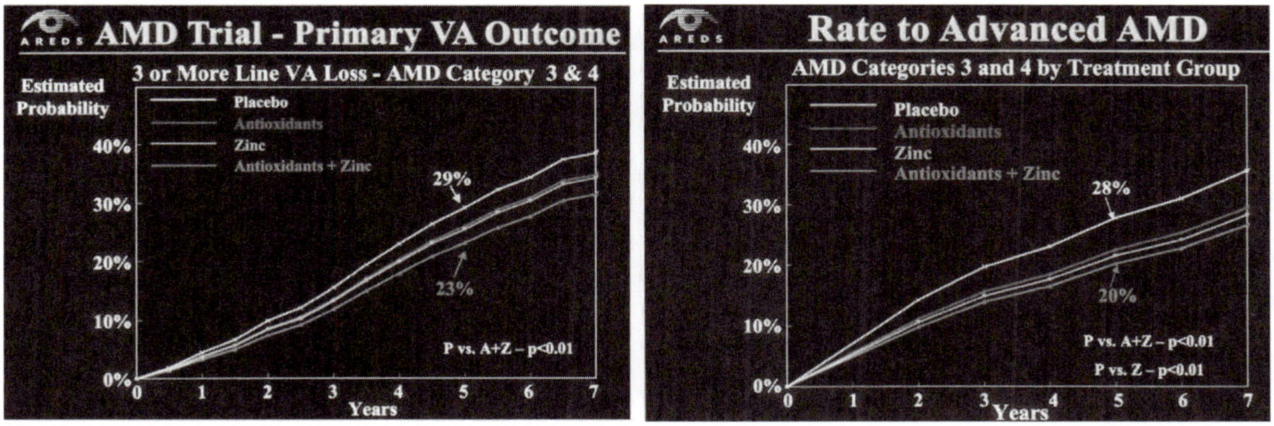

FIGURE 11. (A) Probability of developing visual acuity loss of at least 15 letters in at least one study eye of AREDS participants in AREDS Categories 3 and 4 by treatment group. (AREDS photographs courtesy of F.L. Ferris, MD, National Eye Institute). (B) Probability of developing advanced AMD in at least one eye of AREDS participants according to treatment group.

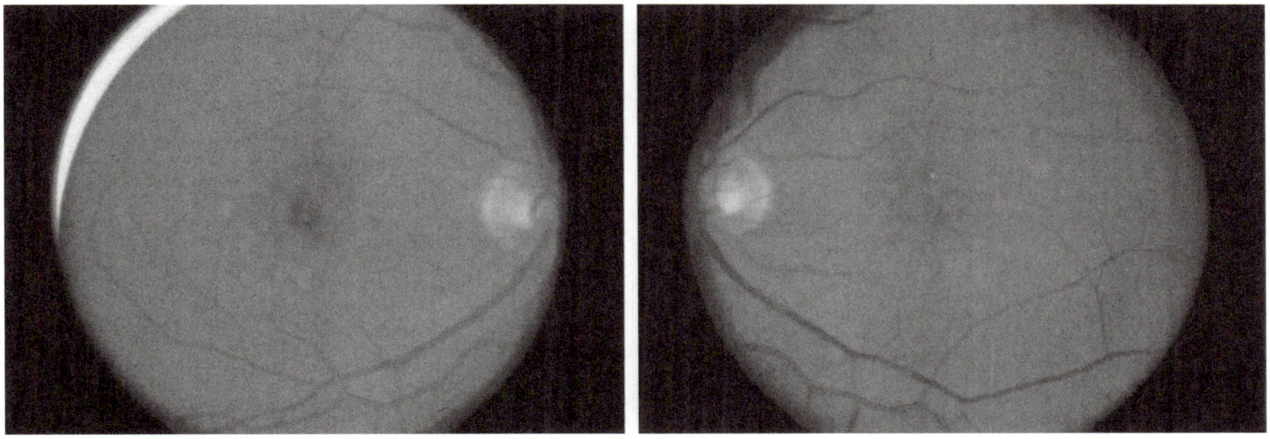

FIGURE 12. Fundus photographs of 60-year-old woman with large, confluent macular drusen in both eyes and a small hemorrhage with lipid exudates in the papillomacular bundle. (A) Right eye. (B) Left eye.

My interest in a trial of preventive laser treatment for eyes with high risk drusen was kindled in 1992. At that time, during a routine follow-up visit, I examined a 60-year-old patient with visual acuity of 20/15 in each eye, large confluent drusen in each macula, and a small hemorrhage accompanied by lipid exudates in the left papillomacular bundle (Figure 12). A fluorescein angiogram showed subtle but definite abnormal fluorescence in the area adjacent to the hemorrhage and exudates (Figure 13). Biomicroscopy showed slight elevation of the retinal pigmented epithelium (RPE) in this area. Because I strongly suspected that this RPE elevation, associated hemorrhage and lipid, and abnormal fluorescence was caused by a small tuft of extrafoveal choroidal neovascularization, I recommended argon laser photocoagulation despite the fact that this was an asymptomatic lesion in an eye with 20/15 visual acuity. The patient agreed with my recommendation, and laser treatment (two overlapping burns) was carried out uneventfully. In a few weeks, the blood disappeared, the RPE flattened, and the laser-induced paracentral scotoma became asymptomatic. Nine months after laser treatment, the drusen in the untreated right eye were still large, confluent, and as numerous as nine months previously, whereas the drusen in the laser-treated left eye had largely disappeared except for a few drusen 180 degrees opposite the area treated with laser (Figure 14). I speculated that the laser application to the small neovascular lesion in the left eye might have promoted resolution of the macular drusen by some unknown mechanism. Several months later, while still pondering this question, I read a report describing 20 patients who showed some resolution of drusen under the fovea and in the nasal portion of the macula after low intensity laser photocoagulation had been applied directly only to drusen located in the temporal portion of the macula.[55] On average, drusen in the temporal macula treated directly with laser disappeared within two months, whereas nasal drusen and foveal drusen, presumably as a result of indirect laser treatment, required

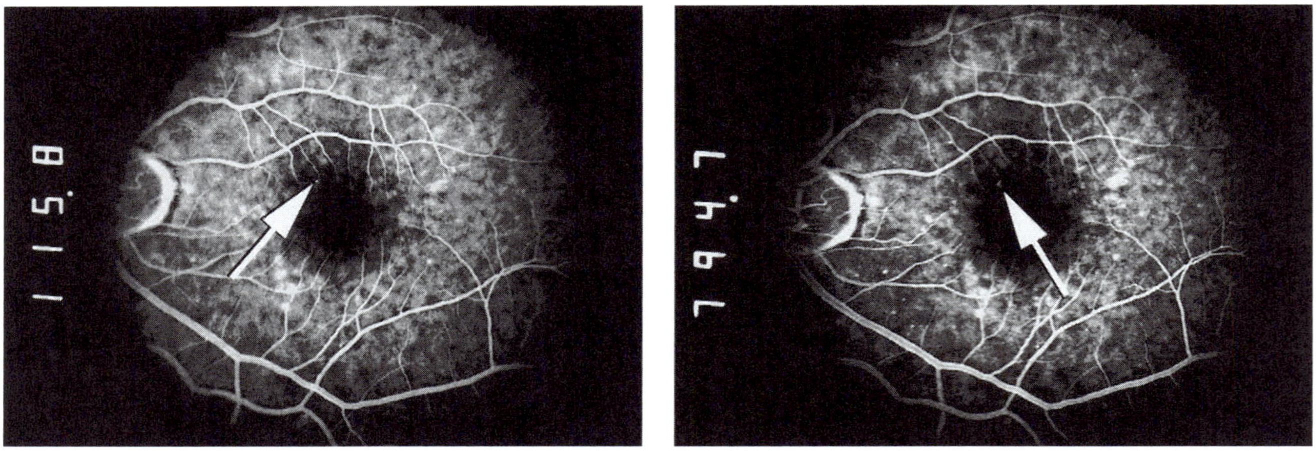

FIGURE 13. Fluorescein angiogram of patient showing subtle but definite hyperfluorescence (arrow) adjacent to macular hemorrhage, left eye. (A) Early phase angiogram. (B) Late phase angiogram

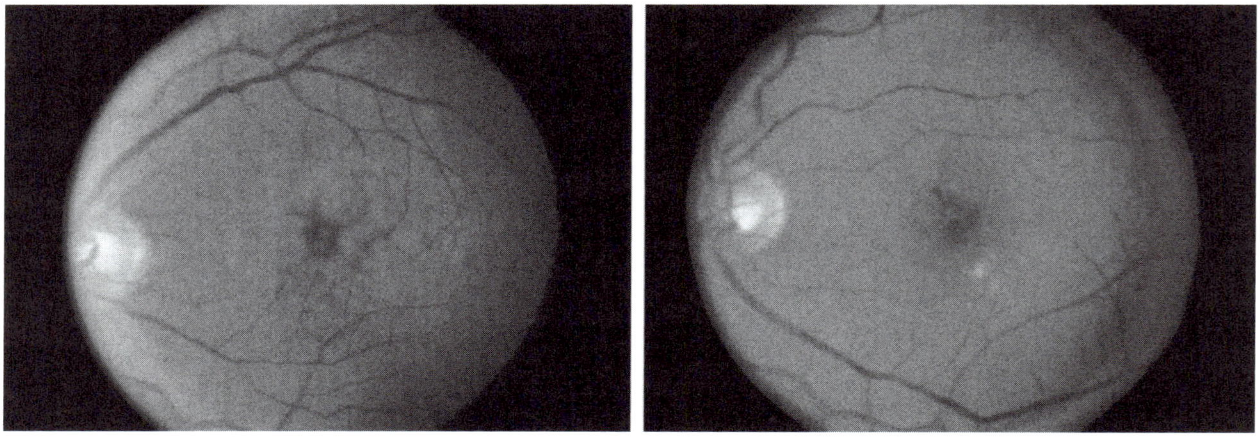

FIGURE 14. Patient illustrated in Figures 13 and 14, nine months following laser photocoagulation to area of presumed choroidal neovascularization in papillomacular bundle of left eye. (A) Right macula (untreated). Compare with Figure 12A. (B) Left macula (laser treated). Compare with Figure 12B.

an average of 10 months for resolution. To investigate further the possible relationship between laser photocoagulation and drusen resolution, the MPS Reading Center evaluated a group of patients who had been treated successfully with laser in their study eyes, who had not developed recurrent leakage in the treated study eye, and who had drusen in the fellow eye. Over a follow-up period of three years, laser treated eyes were far more likely to show drusen resolution than untreated fellow eyes (unpublished data).

There was now information from several sources suggesting that photocoagulation or laser treatment in the macular region was followed by the disappearance of or reduction in the extent of drusen. These data, when considered in the aggregate, provided the impetus to consider a clinical trial to evaluate the ability of low intensity laser treatment, not only to promote drusen resolution but more importantly to reduce the risk of disease progression and its attendant risk of vision loss in eyes with high risk drusen.

My colleague, Dr. Maureen Maguire, Professor of Ophthalmology and Director of the Center for Preventive Ophthalmology and Biostatistics at the Scheie Eye Institute of the University of Pennsylvania, and I proposed a pilot study, the Choroidal Neovascularization Prevention Trial or CNVPT. This trial, consisting of two sub-studies, the Fellow Eye Study and the Bilateral Drusen Study, was conducted at 16 participating clinical centers between 1994 and 1998 (Figure 15). Beginning in 1994, 120 patients enrolled in the Fellow Eye Study, and 156 patients enrolled in the Bilateral Drusen Study. The CNVPT treatment protocol stipulated the placement of a total of 20 relatively low intensity lesions, each 100 microns in diameter, in three concentric arcs temporal to the fovea in the eye assigned to treatment (Figure 16). Six months later, if the eye assigned to laser treatment still would be

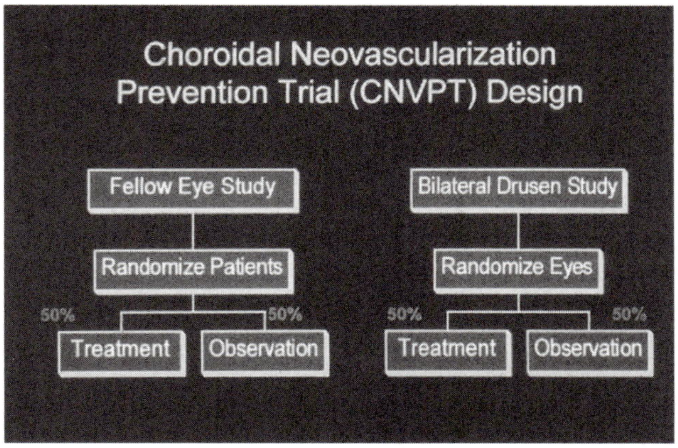

FIGURE 15. Choroidal Neovascularization Prevention Trial Study design for Fellow Eye Study and Bilateral Drusen Study.

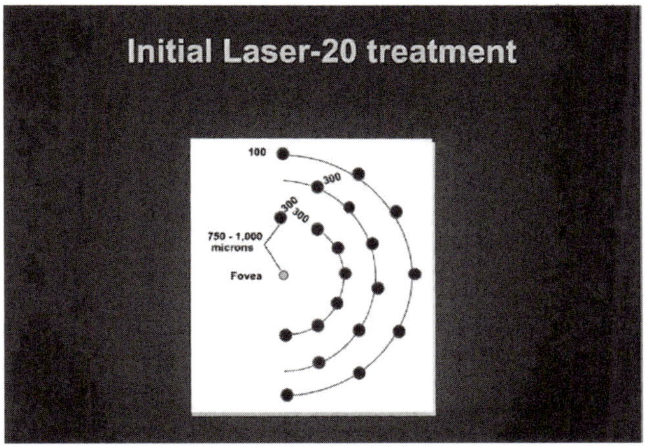

FIGURE 16. Protocol treatment in Choroidal Neovascularization Prevention Trial. Initial laser treatment consists of 20 lesions in three arcs temporal to fovea.

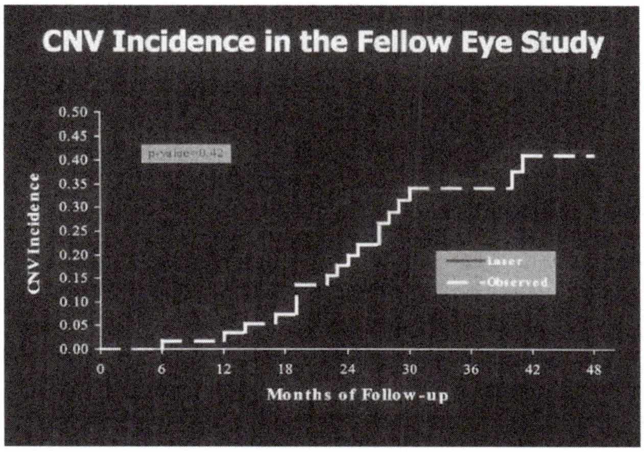

FIGURE 17. Reprinted with permission from Ophthalmol Vol 110, No. 5 p. 974, May 2003. Rates of choroidal neovascularization in CNVPT Fellow Eye Study "Estimated cumulative proportion of eyes developing choroidal neovascularization by treatment group." At no time was there a significant difference in visual outcome in treated fellow eyes vs untreated fellow eyes.

eligible to be enrolled in CNVPT, 20 additional laser lesions were placed in three concentric arcs on the nasal side of the fovea.

Prior to beginning patient enrollment in the CNVPT, Dr. Maguire and I appointed a Data and Safety Monitoring Committee (DSMC) to review the protocol as well as the data that would be accumulating with regard to both safety and possible efficacy. In planning this pilot, it never was intended that a sufficient number of patients would be enrolled to answer the study question definitively with regard to efficacy. While the CNVPT ophthalmologists felt confident from the outset that the protocol laser treatment would promote at least partial resolution of drusen, they also thought that the risk of toxicity from the relatively low intensity laser application required by the study protocol was extremely small, absenting an inadvertent laser burn to the fovea. Thus, the investigators were surprised when the DSMC reported in December 1996, two years after patient enrollment began, that in the Fellow Eye Study only, laser-treated eyes were more likely than observed eyes to have progressed to choroidal neovascularization, the opposite of the anticipated effect of preventive laser treatment (Figure 17). Fortunately, in this group of laser-treated fellow eyes in the Fellow Eye Study, there was no accompanying increase in the frequency of vision loss compared to the group of observed fellow eyes. Nevertheless, on advice from the Data and Safety Monitoring Committee, the CNVPT investigators took the following actions:

- Halt the enrollment of all new patients in both the Fellow Eye Study and the Bilateral Drusen Study
- Inform all patients in both the Fellow Eye Study and Bilateral Drusen Study of this unexpected finding in the Fellow Eye Study
- Halt all preventive laser treatments, including protocol follow-up treatments, in both studies
- Inform the ophthalmic community about this unexpected finding, in an effort to discourage practicing ophthalmologists from performing similar preventive treatments in patients not enrolled in the CNVPT studies[56]
- Follow all patients in the Fellow Eye Study for up to four years

All of the aforementioned recommendations were carried out. By the time patients in the Fellow Eye Study had been followed up for four years, it was clear that, 30 months after enrollment, the rates of choroidal neovascularization in treated eyes and untreated eyes in the Fellow Eye Study were identical (Figure 17).[57]

Among the 156 patients enrolled in the Bilateral Drusen Study, there was never an indication that laser-treated eyes were more likely than untreated eyes to develop choroidal neovascularization. Accordingly, once it became clear that there was no evidence of long term toxicity from low intensity laser treatment in the CNVPT Fellow Eye Study, the investigators again considered the possibility of conducting a definitive trial, sufficiently powered with respect to the number of patients to be enrolled, to determine whether laser treatment could reduce the likelihood of progression from high risk drusen to late AMD and accompanying loss of vision in patients with large, confluent drusen in both eyes.

In designing that definitive trial of preventive laser treatment, we used information learned from the CNVPT and from another trial with a similar study design, the Prophylactic Treatment for Age-Related Macular Degeneration Study (PTAMD), chaired by Dr. Thomas Friberg of the University of Pittsburgh. The information that was used to plan the next trial is summarized below.

(1) The intensity of the laser burn, as applied to eyes with high risk drusen, was positively correlated with the risk of developing CNV in laser treated eyes.[58]
(2) Since eyes with high risk drusen that develop CNV following laser treatment most often exhibit the occult form of CNV, with little or no accompanying vision loss, annual fluorescein angiograms would be necessary to detect the primary endpoint CNV that was often asymptomatic.
(3) A larger number of low intensity laser burns delivered to the macular region was not associated with any significant toxicity and might be more effective in reducing the extent of drusen.

Accordingly, the definitive protocol for the new trial incorporated what had been learned from the CNVPT and from the PTAMD studies.[59] In this new NEI-supported trial, known as the Complications of AMD Prevention Trial (CAPT), the study question is whether, in patients with high risk drusen in both eyes, low intensity laser treatment applied to one eye selected at random, could reduce the risk of vision loss and the risk of progression to either choroidal neovascularization or geographic atrophy. Between 1999 and 2001, the CAPT enrolled 1052 patients at 22 clinical centers (Figure 18). One eye of each patient was assigned randomly to receive the protocol laser treatment (Figure 19A). One year after treatment, patients who had less than 50% reduction in the extent of drusen were eligible for a second protocol laser treatment (Figure 19B) unless they had developed CNV or geographic atrophy in the eye assigned to treatment or CNV in the fellow (untreated) eye. A Data and Safety Monitoring Committee has been meeting at six-month intervals to monitor the effects of treatment with respect to safety and efficacy. At its most recent meeting, in April 2004, the DSMC confirmed that the CAPT study is sufficiently powered to provide an answer concerning the efficacy of the intervention under study by the anticipated study closing date in the spring of 2006. The PTAMD study expects to have outcome data available within the same time frame.

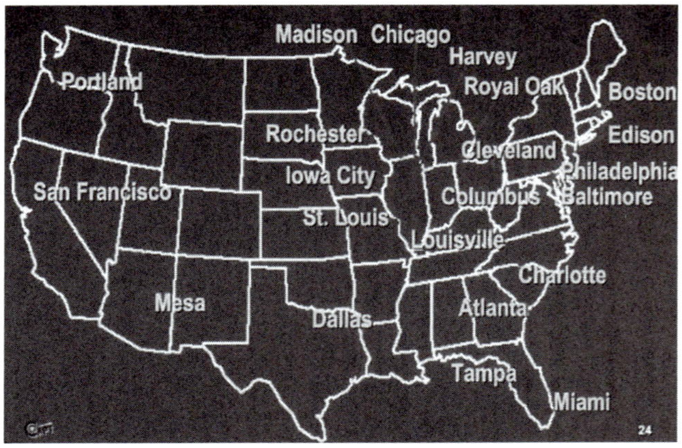

FIGURE 18. Location of 22 clinical centers participating in Complications of AMD Prevention Trial which is supported by the National Eye Institute.

In the meantime, several ongoing analyses of CAPT patients already have been reported. Stoltz and associates reported that drusen remodeling, pigmentary alterations, and foveal atrophy which does not achieve the CAPT criteria for a diagnosis of geographic atrophy are responsible for most vision loss of ≥ three but ≤ six lines on an ETDRS chart. (Stoltz RA, et al. Fundus features of untreated eyes with visual acuity loss in CAPT. April 26, 2004 presentation at ARVO. IOVS 1389, B200). Alexander and associates have confirmed that most of the CNV which occurs is of the occult type. (Alexander J, et al. Characteristics of exudation in patients with bilateral large drusen. April 27, 2004 presentation at ARVO. IOVS 2989, B624).

Of more than passing interest is a recent publication from Sweden which reported that in a randomized pilot study involving 38 patients with soft drusen maculopathy, preventive laser treatment reduced the rate of exudative complications to a statistically significant degree. However, because of the small sample size and despite eight years of follow-up, the authors urged caution in the interpretation of the results.[60]

A pharmacologic intervention, recently launched, is evaluating whether juxtascleral anecortave acetate, compared to sham injection, can reduce the rate of progression from extensive drusen and pigment clumping to neovascularization in the second eye of patients who already have lost vision from late AMD in the first eye. Anecortave acetate is thought to work by inhibiting the action of cellular proteases that are needed for the migration of vascular endothelial cells. In a 12-month Phase II trial involving 128 patients, treated eyes were less likely to experience vision loss than untreated eyes.[61] Recruitment of over 500 patients was completed in August 2003 for a Phase III trial of anecortave acetate vs PDT for predominantly classic subfoveal CNV. Twelve-month outcome

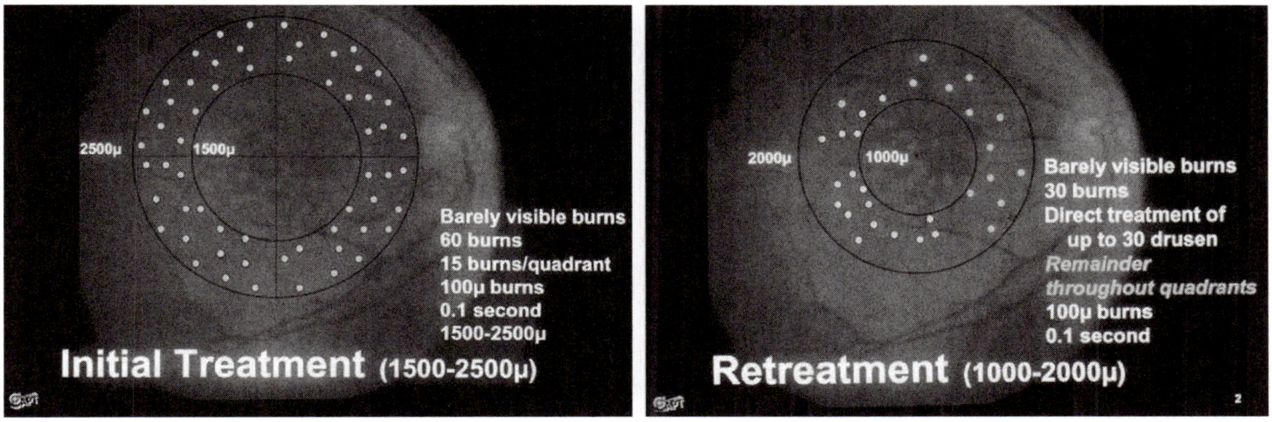

FIGURE 19. Protocol laser treatment for Complications of AMD Prevention Trial (CAPT). (A) Initial laser treatment protocol. (B) Follow-up treatment protocol at one year.

TABLE 3. Important Features of Clinical Trials

- Accurate description of disease
- Understanding natural history
- Well defined treatment protocol
- Adequate sample size
- Informed consent by eligible study participants
- Controls achieved by randomization
- Appropriate length of follow up
- Biometric data analysis
- Independent data and safety monitoring committee

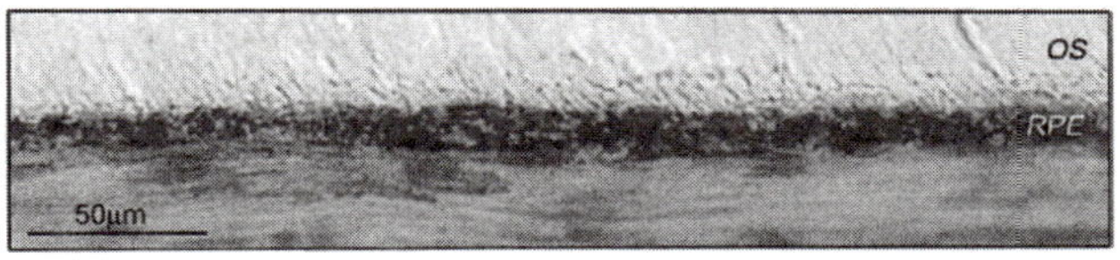

FIGURE 20. Perls' stain (blue) shows iron overload in the retinal pigment epithelium in ceruloplasmin/hephaestin deficient mice.

data were reported by Carl Regillo at the pre-Academy Retina Subspecialty Day meeting on October 22, 2004.

During the fourth era, which begins in 2004, several ongoing trials will be completed and the results with indications for patient care will be published. Recently, the Submacular Surgery Trials Group reported that submacular surgery in eligible AMD patients did not improve the overall chance for stable or improved visual acuity compared to observation.[62,63] More detailed analyses may identify one or more subgroups that derive a benefit from this intervention. During the next decade, I expect that the role of anti-VEGF therapy, including combination therapy, will be sorted out by means of clinical trials (Table 3). I expect that prevention trials will be conducted for patients with very early AMD. I expect that new information, being developed in laboratories around the world, will shed light on the pathogenesis of AMD. Hahn and associates have found that AMD retinas exhibit iron overload.[64] While this finding does not prove that iron overload is a cause of AMD, several additional findings from that laboratory support this possibility. First, a line of mice with retinal iron overload attributable to mutations in the iron transporters, ceruloplasmin and hephaestin, develop some features of AMD, including neovascularization in the subretinal space.[65] Second, a patient with the rare autosomal recessive disease, aceruloplasminemia, which results in retinal iron overload, developed drusen at the young age of 47 (Dunaief JL, written communication, August 19, 2004). Third, ceruloplasmin is upregulated in mouse retinas exposed to photo-oxidative stress, possibly as a defense against iron induced oxidative stress.[66] Dunaief's lab is now testing whether an iron chelating agent can reduce the retinal iron overload in the ceruloplasmin/hephaestin deficient mice (Figure 20). If so, could iron chelation become another non-surgical intervention for AMD?

Another recent finding, that of amyloid-beta in drusen, first reported in Anderson's lab and subsequently confirmed by Dunaief's lab, suggests that drusen may have some features of extracellular plaques found in Alzheimer's Disease brains (Figure 21).[67,68] A potential link between the pathogenesis of AMD and Alzheimer's Disease suggests that anti-amyloid-beta therapies under development for Alzheimer's may prove useful for AMD.

In looking to the future, other lines of investigation include creating animal models for both drusen and choroidal neovascularization by overexpression of certain genes, and exploring the role of genetics, altered blood flow, inflammation, and the role of PEDF and growth factors other than VEGF. Remarkably, psychophysicists now can detect subtle disturbances in macular function before there are visible macular abnormalities. If nontoxic interventions are shown to be of value in presymptomatic patients, these psychophysical assessments could identify the subjects who should be evaluated. Once effective

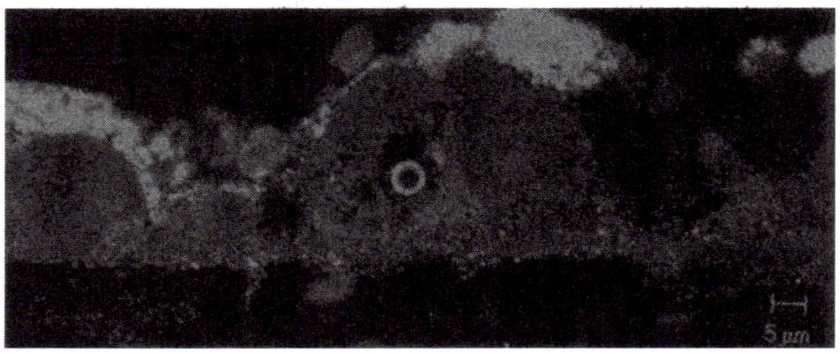

FIGURE 21. Figure reprinted with permission from Molecular Vision, September 2003; Vol 9, p. 188. Photomicrograph shows that anti-amyloid-beta-antibody 2332 detects a single vesicle and punctuate granular deposits within drusen.

pharmacologic treatment becomes available, the next hurdle will be to develop a delivery system which ideally would not require repeated retrobulbar, periocular, or intravitreal injections. An effective treatment delivered as an eye drop or through a slow release polymer injected into the vitreous cavity would be a significant advantage over routes of administration currently employed in most ongoing eye trials.

During my 35 years in ophthalmology, AMD has moved from the rear balcony to center stage. In 1969, when I first heard the term senile macular degeneration from my University of Florida mentor, Dr. Melvin Rubin, I had to look it up. The Framingham Eye Study had not yet issued its first report on the prevalence of AMD as a cause of vision loss. But despite the plethora of trials and the emergence of treatments of some value, AMD remains the major cause of severe and irreversible vision loss in the United States and throughout the developed world. Each year, 200,000 AMD patients in the United States develop choroidal neovascularization and that number will rise considerably as the population ages, absent the introduction of one or more highly effective interventions.[69,70] Thus AMD remains the greatest unsolved problem in ophthalmology in the developed world. On the positive side is the enormous interest of the National Eye Institute, large pharmaceutical companies, and the many investigators actively conducting research. These endeavors, and the emphasis on prevention trials, provide much hope for the future. In the meantime, we must acknowledge our current limitations in treating AMD patients and remember that low vision rehabilitation, treatment for depression, when appropriate, and the empathetic ophthalmologist are crucial components of patient care. My fervent wish is that the next Jackson lecturer who selects AMD as a topic will describe the quantifiable benefits of a highly effective treatment that is broadly applicable to the universe of patients at risk for vision loss from AMD. In the meantime, the honor of this Edward Jackson Memorial lectureship is dedicated to all the patients still suffering from AMD and to all the investigators laboring to find better treatments. With their continued efforts, AMD may no longer be the scourge of the elderly.

REFERENCES

1. Gass JDM. Pathogenesis of disciform detachment of the neuroepithelium. IV. Fluorescein angiographic study of senile disciform macular degeneration. Am J Ophthalmol 1967;63:617–645.
2. Leibowitz HM, Krueger DE, Maunder RA, et al. The Framingham Eye Study monograph: an ophthalmological and epidemiological study of cataract, glaucoma, diabetic retinopathy, macular degeneration, and visual acuity in a general population of 2631 adults, 1973–1975. Surv Ophthalmol 1980;24(suppl):335–610.
3. Hyman LG, Lilienfeld AM, Ferris FL, Fine SL, et al. Senile macular degeneration: a case-control study. Am J Epidemiol 1983;118:213–227.
4. Bressler NM, et al. The grading and prevalence of macular degeneration in Chesapeake Bay watermen. Arch Ophthalmol 1989;107:847–852.
5. Klein R, et al. The relationship of age-related maculopathy, cataract, and glaucoma to visual acuity. Invest Ophthalmol Vis Sci 1995;36:182–191.
6. Klein R, Klein BEK, Moss SE. Relation of smoking to the incidence of age-related maculopathy: the Beaver Dam Eye Study. Am J Epidemiol 1998;147:103–110.
7. Klein R, Klein BEK, Franke T. The relationship of cardiovascular disease and its risk factors to age-related maculopathy: the Beaver Dam Eye Study. Ophthalmology 1993;100: 406–414.
8. Klein R, Klein BEK, Jensen SC. The relation of cardiovascular disease and its risk factors to the 5 year incidence of age-related maculopathy: the Beaver Dam Eye Study. Ophthalmology 1997;104:1804–1812.
9. Mitchell P, Smith W, Attebo K, Wang JJ, et al. Prevalence of age-related maculopathy in Australia: the Blue Mountains Eye Study. Ophthalmology 1995;102:2450–1460.
10. Vingerling JR, Hofman A, Diederick E, et al. Age-related macular degeneration and smoking: the Rotterdam Study. Arch Ophthalmol 1996;114:1193–1196.
11. Vinding T, et al. Risk factor analysis for atrophic and exudative age-related macular degeneration: an epidemiological study of 1000 aged individuals. Acta Ophthalmol (Copenh) 1992;70:66–72.
12. Eye Disease Case-Control Study Group. Risk factors for neovascular age-related macular degeneration, Arch Ophthalmol 1992;110:1701–1708.
13. Eye Disease Case-Control Study Group. Risk factors for neovascular age-related macular degeneration, Arch Ophthalmol 1992;110:1701–1708.
14. West SK, Rosenthal SF, Bressler NM, et al. Exposure to sunlight and other risk factors for age-related macular degeneration. Arch Ophthalmol 1989;107:875–879.
15. Seddon JM, Willett WC, Speizer FE, Hankinson SE, et al. A prospective study of cigarette smoking and age-related macular degeneration in women. JAMA 1996;276:1141–1146.

16. Christen WG, Glynn RJ, Manson JE, et al. A prospective study of cigarette smoking and risk of age-related macular degeneration in men. JAMA 1996;276:1147–1151.
17. Diabetic retinopathy Study Research Group. Preliminary report on effects of photocoagulation therapy. Am J Ophthalmol 1976;81:383–396.
18. Patz A, Hoeck LE, De la Cruz E. Studies on the effect of high oxygen administration in retrolental fibroplasias. I. Nursery observations. Am J Ophthalmol 1952;35:1248–1253.
19. Patz A. Oxygen studies in retrolental fibroplasias. IV. Clinical and experimental observations. Am J Ophthalmol 1954; 38:291–308.
20. Moorfields Macular Study Group. Treatment of senile disciform macular degeneration: a single-blind randomized trial by argon laser photocoagulation. Brit. J Ophthalmol 1982; 66:745–753.
21. Coscas G, Soubrane G. Photocoagulation des neo vaisseaux sous-retiniens dans la degenerescence maculaire senile par laser a argon: resultants de letude randomisee de 60 cas. Bull Mem Soc Fr Ophtalmol 1982;94:149–154.
22. Macular Photocoagulation Study Group. Argon laser photocoagulation for senile macular degeneration. Results of a randomized clinical trial. Arch Ophthalmol 1982;100:912–918.
23. Macular Photocoagulation Study Group. Krypton laser photocoagulation for neovascular lesions of age-related macular degeneration. Results of a randomized clinical trial. Arch Ophthalmol 1990;108:816–824
24. Schatz H, Yannuzzi LA, Gitter KA. Subretinal neovascularization following argon laser photocoagulation treatment for central serous chorioretinopathy: complication or misdiagnosis? Trans Am Acad Ophthalmol Otolaryngol 1977;83: 893–906.
25. Ryan SJ. Subretinal neovascularization. Natural history of an experimental model. Arch Ophthalmol 1982;100:1804–1809.
26. Yannuzzi LA, Slakter JS, Sorensen JA, Guyer DR, Orlock DA, et al. Digital indocyanine green video-angiography of occult choroidal neovascularization. Retina 1992;12:191–223.
27. Schuman JS, Puliafito CA, Fujimoto JG, et al. Optical coherence tomography of ocular diseases. Thorofare: SLACK, 1996.
28. Bird AC, Bressler NM, Bressler SM, et al. An International ARM Epidemiology Study Group. An international classification and grading system for age-related maculopathy and age-related macular degeneration. Survey Ophthalmol 1995; 39:367–374.
29. Macular Photocoagulation Study Group. Subfoveal neovascular lesions in age-related macular degeneration. Arch Ophthalmol 1991;109:1242–1257
30. Bressler SB, Bressler NM, Fine SL, et al. Natural course of choroidal neovascular membranes within the foveal avascular zone in senile macular degeneration. Am J Ophthalmol 1982;93:157–163
31. Guyer DR, Fine SL, Maguire MG, Hawkins BS, Owens SL, Murphy RP. Subfoveal neovascular membranes in age-related macular degeneration: visual prognosis in eyes with relatively good initial visual acuity. Arch Ophthalmol 1986; 104:702–705.
32. Macular Photocoagulation Study Group. Argon laser photocoagulation for neovascular maculopathy. Arch Ophthalmol 1991;109:1109–1111
33. Jampol LM. Hypertension and visual outcome in the Macula Photocoagulation Study. Arch Ophthalmol 1991;109(6): 789–790.
34. Macular Photocoagulation Study Group. Laser photocoagulation of subfoveal recurrent neovascular lesion in age-related macular degeneration. Results of randomized clinical trial. Arch Ophthalmol 1991;109:1220–1231.
35. Macular Photocoagulation Study Group. Laser photocoagulation of subfoveal neovascular lesions in age-related macular degeneration. Results of a randomized clinical trial. Arch Ophthalmol 1991;109:1232–1241.
36. Macular Photocoagulation Study Group. Visual outcome after laser photocoagulation for subfoveal choroidal neovascularization secondary to age-related macular degeneration. The influence of initial lesion size and initial visual acuity. Arch Ophthalmol 1994;112:480–488.
37. Strahlman ER, Fine SL, Hillis A. The second eye of patients with senile macular degeneration. Arch Ophthalmol 1984; 91:271–277.
38. Macular Photocoagulation Study Group. Risk factors for choroidal neovascularization in the second eye of patients with juxtafoveal or subfoveal choroidal neovascularization secondary to age-related macular degeneration. Arch Ophthalmol 1997;115:741–747.
39. Smiddy WE, Fine SL. Prognosis of patients with bilateral macular drusen. Ophthalmology 1984;91:271–277.
40. Holz FG, Wolfensberger TJ, Piguet B, et al. Bilateral macular drusen in age-related macular degeneration. Ophthalmology 1994;101:1522–1528.
41. D'Amato RJ, Loughnan MS, Flynn E, Folkman J. Thalidomide is an inhibitor of angiogenesis. Proc Natl Acad Sci USA 1994;91:4082–4085.
42. Pharmacological Therapy for Macular Degeneration Study Group. Interferon alfa-2a is ineffective for patients with choroidal neovascularization secondary to age-related macular degeneration. Results of a prospective randomized placebo-controlled clinical trial. Arch Ophthalmol 1997;115: 865–872.
43. Chakravarthy U, Gardiner TA, Archer DB, Maguire CJ. A light microscopic and autoradiographic study of non-irradiated and irradiated ocular wounds. Current Eye Res 1989;8: 337–348.
44. Chakravarthy U, Houston RF, Archer DB. Treatment of age-related subfoveal neovascular membranes by teletherapy: a pilot study. Br J Ophthalmol 1993;77:261–262.
45. Radiation Therapy for Neovascular Age-Related Macular Degeneration Research Group. A prospective, randomized, double-masked trial on radiation therapy for neovascular age-related macular degeneration (RAD Study). Ophthalmology 1999;106:2239–2247.
46. Fine SL, Maguire MG. It is not time to abandon radiotherapy for neovascular age-related macular degeneration. Arch Ophthalmol 2001;119:275–276.
47. Age-Related Macular Degeneration and Radiotherapy Trial Research Group. The Age-related macular degeneration radiotherapy trial (AMDRT): One year results from a pilot study. Am J Ophthalmol 2004;5;818–828.
48. Treatment of Age-Related Macular Degeneration with Photodynamic Therapy (TAP) Study Group. Photodynamic therapy of subfoveal choroidal neovascularization in age-

related macular degeneration with verteporfin. Arch Ophthalmol 1999;117:1329–1345.
49. Miller JW, Schmidt-Erfurth U, Sickenberg M, et al. Photodynamic therapy with verteporfin for choroidal neovascularization caused by age-related macular degeneration: results of a single treatment in a phase 1 and 2 study. Arch Ophthalmol 1999;117:1161–1173.
50. Schmidt-Erfurth U, Miller JW, Sickenberg M, et al. Photodynamic therapy with verteporfin for choroidal neovascularization caused by age-related macular degeneration: results of retreatments in a phase 1 and 2 study. Arch Ophthalmol 1999;117:1177–1187.
51. Verteporfin in Photodynamic Therapy Study Group. Verteporfin therapy of subfoveal choroidal neovascularization in age-related macular degeneration: two-year results of a randomized, clinical trial including lesions with occult with no classic choroidal neovascularization-Verteporfin in photodynamic therapy report 2. Am J Ophthalmol 2001;131:541–560.
52. Treatment of Age-Related Macular Degeneration with Photodynamic Therapy and Verteporfin in Photodynamic Therapy Study Groups. Effect of lesion size, visual acuity, and lesion composition on visual acuity change with and without verteporfin therapy for choroidal neovascularization secondary to age-related macular degeneration: TAP and VIP report No. 1. Am J Ophthalmol 2003;136:407–418.
53. Lanconey DM, Maguire MG, Fine SL. A model of incidence and consequences of choroidal neovascularization secondary to age-related macular degeneration. Arch Ophthalmol 1998;116:1045–1052.
54. Age-Related Eye Disease Study Research Group. AREDS Report #8. A randomized, placebo-controlled, clinical trial of high-dose supplementation with vitamins C and E, beta carotene, and zinc for age-related macular degeneration and vision loss. Arch Ophthalmol 2001;119:1417–1436.
55. Figueroa MS, Regueras A, Bertrand J. Laser photocoagulation to treat macular soft drusen in age-related macular degeneration. Retina 1994;14:391–396.
56. Choroidal Neovascularization Prevention Trial Research Group. Laser treatment in eyes with large drusen: short term effects from a pilot randomized clinical trial. Ophthalmology 1998;105:11–23.
57. Choroidal Neovascularization Prevention Trial Research Group. Laser treatment in fellow eyes with large drusen: updated findings from a pilot randomized clinical trial. Ophthalmology 2003;110:971–978.
58. Kaiser RS, Berger JW, Maguire MG, Ho AC, Javornik NB, Choroidal Neovascularization Prevention Trial (CNVPT) Study Group. Laser burn intensity and the risk of choroidal neovascularization in the CMVPT Fellow Eye Study. Arch Ophthalmol 2001;119:826–832.
59. Rodanant N, Friberg TR, Cheng L, et al. Predictors of drusen reduction after subthreshold infrared (810 nm) diode laser macular grid photocoagulation for nonexudative age-related macular degeneration. Am J Ophthalmol 2002;134:577–585.
60. Frennesson CI. Prophylactic laser treatment in early age-related macular degeneration: an 8-year follow-up in a randomized pilot study shows a reduced incidence of exudative complications. Acta Ophthalmologica Scandinavica 2003;81:449–454.
61. D'Amico DJ, Goldberg MF, Hudson H, et al. Anecortave acetate as monotherapy for treatment of subfoveal neovascularization in age-related macular degeneration: twelve-month clinical outcomes. Ophthalmology 2003;110:2372–2383.
62. Submacular Surgery Trials Research Group. Surgery for subfoveal choroidal neovascularization in age-related macular degeneration: Ophthalmic findings. SST Report No. 11. Ophthalmology 2004;111:1967–1980.
63. Submacular Surgery Trials Research Group. Surgery for hemorrhagic choroidal neovascular lesions of age-related macular degeneration: Ophthalmic findings. SST Report No. 13. Ophthalmology 2004;111:1993–2006.
64. Hahn P, Milam AH, Dunaief JL. Maculas affected by age-related macular degeneration contain increased chelatable iron in the retinal pigment epithelium and Bruch's membrane. Arch Ophthalmol 2003;121:1099–1105.
65. Hahn P, Ying Q, Dentchev T, et al. Disruption of ceruloplasmin and hephaestin in mice causes retinal iron overload and retinal degeneration with features of age-related macular degeneration. Proc Natl Acad Sci USA 2004;101(38):13850–13855.
66. Chen L, Dentchev T, Wong R, Wen R, Bennett J, Dunaief JL. Increased expression of ceruloplasmin in the retina following photic injury. Mol Vis 2003;30:151–158.
67. Johnson LV, Leitner WP, Rivest AJ, Staples MK, Radeke MJ, Anderson DH. The Alzheimer's A beta-peptide is deposited at sites of complement activation in pathologic deposits associated with aging and age-related macular degeneration. Proc Natl Acad Sci USA 2002;99:11830–11835.
68. Dentchev T, Milam AH, Lee VM, Trojanowski JQ, Dunaief JL. Amyloid-beta is found in drusen from some age-related macular degeneration retinas, but not in drusen from normal retinas. Mol Vis 2003;14:9184–9190.
69. The Eye Disease Prevalence Research Group. Causes and prevalence of visual impairment among adults in the United States. Arch Ophthalmol 2004;122:477–485.
70. Incidence of age-related macular degeneration among elderly Americans. Ophthalmology 2003;110:1534–1539.

NOTES

NOTES

NOTES

ISBN 1-933087-34-X
ISSN 1542-1961
Printed in the United States of America

JOHNS HOPKINS
MEDICINE

The Johns Hopkins White Papers are published yearly by Medletter Associates, LLC.

Visit our website for information on Johns Hopkins Health Publications, which include White Papers on specific disorders, home medical encyclopedias, consumer reference guides to drugs and medical tests, and our monthly newsletter *The Johns Hopkins Medical Letter: Health After 50*.
www.JohnsHopkinsHealthAlerts.com

JOHNS HOPKINS MEDICINE

The 2006 White Papers

66AWHP

Take Control of Your Medical Condition

Visit us online at www.JohnsHopkinsHealthAlerts.com/bookstore

YES, I've placed a check mark next to the White Paper(s) I'd like to receive for $19.95 each. Annual updates on each subject that I have chosen will be offered to me by announcement card. I need do nothing if I want the update to be sent to me automatically. If I do not want it, I will return the announcement card marked "cancel." I may cancel at any time. (Please add $2.95 for domestic, $4.95 for Canadian, and $15.00 for foreign orders to your total to cover shipping and handling.) (CT, FL, IL, MA and OH residents add sales tax.)

✔ Please put a check mark next to the White Paper(s) you wish to order.

001065	❑ Arthritis	$19.95
003061	❑ Coronary Heart Disease	$19.95
004069	❑ Depression and Anxiety	$19.95
005066	❑ Diabetes	$19.95
006064	❑ Hypertension and Stroke	$19.95
007062	❑ Nutrition and Weight Control for Longevity	$19.95
008060	❑ Prostate Disorders	$19.95
010066	❑ Digestive Disorders	$19.95
011064	❑ Vision	$19.95
012062	❑ Back Pain & Osteoporosis	$19.95
015065	❑ Memory	$19.95
019067	❑ Lung Disorders	$19.95
020065	❑ Heart Attack Prevention	$19.95

Name

Address

City State Zip

METHOD OF PAYMENT: (U.S. funds only) ❑ VISA ❑ MasterCard ❑ Check Enclosed ❑ Bill Me

Credit Card # Exp. Date

Signature Date

Money Back Guarantee: If for any reason, you are not satisfied after receipt of your publications, return your purchase within 30 days for a full refund.

Detach and mail this card back to The Johns Hopkins White Papers, P.O. Box 420083, Palm Coast, FL 32142

JOHNS HOPKINS MEDICINE

The 2006 White Papers

66AWHP

Take Control of Your Medical Condition

Visit us online at www.JohnsHopkinsHealthAlerts.com/bookstore

YES, I've placed a check mark next to the White Paper(s) I'd like to receive for $19.95 each. Annual updates on each subject that I have chosen will be offered to me by announcement card. I need do nothing if I want the update to be sent to me automatically. If I do not want it, I will return the announcement card marked "cancel." I may cancel at any time. (Please add $2.95 for domestic, $4.95 for Canadian, and $15.00 for foreign orders to your total to cover shipping and handling.) (CT, FL, IL, MA and OH residents add sales tax.)

✔ Please put a check mark next to the White Paper(s) you wish to order.

001065 ❑ Arthritis $19.95
003061 ❑ Coronary Heart Disease $19.95
004069 ❑ Depression and Anxiety $19.95
005066 ❑ Diabetes $19.95
006064 ❑ Hypertension and Stroke $19.95
007062 ❑ Nutrition and Weight Control for Longevity $19.95
008060 ❑ Prostate Disorders $19.95
010066 ❑ Digestive Disorders $19.95
011064 ❑ Vision $19.95
012062 ❑ Back Pain & Osteoporosis $19.95
015065 ❑ Memory $19.95
019067 ❑ Lung Disorders $19.95
020065 ❑ Heart Attack Prevention $19.95

Name

Address

City State Zip

METHOD OF PAYMENT: (U.S. funds only) ❑ VISA ❑ MasterCard ❑ Check Enclosed ❑ Bill Me

Credit Card # Exp. Date

Signature Date

Money Back Guarantee: If for any reason, you are not satisfied after receipt of your publications, return your purchase within 30 days for a full refund.

Detach and mail this card back to The Johns Hopkins White Papers, P.O. Box 420083, Palm Coast, FL 32142

Johns Hopkins White Papers

Fold along this line and tape closed

NO POSTAGE
NECESSARY
IF MAILED
IN THE
UNITED STATES

BUSINESS REPLY MAIL
FIRST-CLASS MAIL PERMIT NO. 86 FLAGLER BEACH FL

POSTAGE WILL BE PAID BY ADDRESSEE

THE JOHNS HOPKINS WHITE PAPERS
PO BOX 420083
PALM COAST FL 32142-9264

Johns Hopkins White Papers

Fold along this line and tape closed

NO POSTAGE
NECESSARY
IF MAILED
IN THE
UNITED STATES

BUSINESS REPLY MAIL
FIRST-CLASS MAIL PERMIT NO. 86 FLAGLER BEACH FL

POSTAGE WILL BE PAID BY ADDRESSEE

THE JOHNS HOPKINS WHITE PAPERS
PO BOX 420083
PALM COAST FL 32142-9264

2006 WHITE PAPER TITLES

ARTHRITIS 2006 - Covers the three most common forms of arthritis–osteoarthritis, rheumatoid arthritis, and gout - as well as two other rheumatic diseases: fibromyalgia syndrome and bursitis.

CORONARY HEART DISEASE 2006 - Discusses four problems resulting from coronary heart disease: angina, heart attacks, heart failure and cardiac arrhythmias.

DEPRESSION and ANXIETY 2006 - Includes major depression, dysthymia, atypical depression, bipolar disorder, seasonal affective disorder, panic disorder, generalized anxiety disorder, obsessive–compulsive disorder, post-traumatic stress disorder, and phobic disorders.

DIABETES 2006 - Shows you how to manage your diabetes and avoid complications such as foot problems and vision changes. Reviews the latest tools for monitoring your blood glucose and the newest medications for controlling it.

DIGESTIVE DISORDERS 2006 - Covers gastroesophageal reflux disease, peptic ulcers, dysphagia, achalasia, Barrett's esophagus, esophageal spasm and stricture, gastritis, gallstones, diarrhea, celiac disease, constipation, Crohn's disease, ulcerative colitis, and colon cancer.

HYPERTENSION and STROKE 2006 - Explains how to treat your high blood pressure and prevent it from harming your health. Also covers the two forms of stroke: ischemic stroke and hemorrhagic stroke.

BACK PAIN and OSTEOPOROSIS 2006 - Addresses back pain due to sprains, strains, and spasms; degenerative changes of the spinal bones and disks; disk herniation; and spinal stenosis. Also covers osteoporosis, a common cause of fractures in the spine and hip.

LUNG DISORDERS 2006 - Includes information on emphysema and chronic bronchitis (together referred to as chronic obstructive pulmonary disease or COPD), asthma, pneumonia, lung cancer, and sleep apnea.

MEMORY 2006 - Tells you how to keep your memory sharp as you get older and how to recognize the symptoms of age-associated memory impairment, mild cognitive impairment, and illnesses such as Alzheimer's disease and vascular dementia.

NUTRITION and WEIGHT CONTROL for LONGEVITY 2006 - Gives you the information you need to eat a healthy diet and keep your weight under control. Also explains what to do when the pounds just don't seem to budge.

PROSTATE DISORDERS 2006 - Helps you decide among the various treatment options for prostate cancer, benign prostatic hyperplasia, and prostatitis.

VISION 2006 - Reviews the current knowledge on cataracts, glaucoma, age-related macular degeneration, and diabetic retinopathy. Also discusses ways to cope with low vision.

HEART ATTACK PREVENTION 2006 - Provides up-to-date strategies for preventing a first heart attack, including identifying possible risk factors, the latest screening tests, risk-reducing lifestyle measures, and medications for controlling cholesterol.